Contents

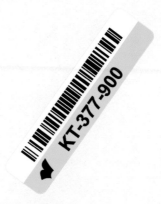

Foreword to the First Edition

The past ten years have seen a steady growth in the number of nurses employed by general practitioners to work in surgery treatment rooms. The wide range of skills required of nurses undertaking such work effectively prompted the Steering Group, established to consider 'The Training Needs of the Practice Nurse', to recommend that these nurses should in future receive recognised training for their role.

This book is, therefore, a welcome and timely publication, not just for the new recruit to practice nursing, but for the established practice nurse intent upon developing the role further, particularly in the field of anticipatory care as considered in the Royal College of General Practitioners Report 'Promoting Prevention'.

The book covers the whole range of knowledge and skills required by a practice nurse during the course of the day-to-day activities in a treatment room. In addition to containing useful chapters on the organisation of general practice and the nurse and the law it offers a very practical guide on equipping a treatment room. A great strength of the book for many practice nurses will be the chapters on nursing procedures, not only because of the attention to detail but for the variety of procedures particularly relevant to the general practice setting which are included.

The clear exposition of the role and function of the practice nurse should enhance professional awareness of the contribution which a nurse makes within the setting of general practice, as should acknowledgement of the part played by the practice nurse alongside that of general practitioner, district nurse and health visitor colleagues within the primary health care team.

Keith Bolden and Beryl Takle, the authors, write with knowledge and understanding of practice nurses and their training needs. This book is published at an opportune moment and should become essential reading, both as a textbook for those in training and a reference book for those already in practice. It should find a place on the shelves of nursing libraries and become a standard text for use by practice nurses.

Annia Fawcett-Henesy

Preface to the Second Edition

Since this book was first written five years ago there have been tremendous developments in both the clinical and medico political fields for practice nurses. Their role is now well established and this book has been revised and rewritten to take account of the many exciting changes which have occurred and to look at the present areas of development.

We hope that those attending training courses for practice nurses will find this book particularly helpful.

Keith J. Bolden
Beryl A. Takle

Chapter 1

The Practice Nurse

The term *practice nurse* is now generally applied to that person who is a Registered General (formerly a State Registered) Nurse employed by a general practitioner and working within the treatment room of the practice. This implication may well be correct for many nurses who consider themselves to be the practice nurse. However, there will be quite a number of other nurses who would also feel that they qualify for this title. They would include Enrolled Nurses (General) (formerly State Enrolled Nurses), community nurses who spend some time in the day working in treatment rooms, and some nurses whose role has become so expanded that they almost, or do, qualify for the title of nurse practitioner.

It is because the role is so undefined and other terms such as *treatment room nurse* are also used that some confusion still exists about who the practice nurse is, when the term is used, and also what her qualification and experience will be.

What is certain is that, far from being a dying breed, the nurses who work within the practice are steadily increasing in number and are exerting pressure on nursing colleagues and the medical profession to recognise their special skills and needs, which are different from those of their colleagues working entirely in a hospital setting or the community. Practice nurses are usually about the age of forty, have married and had a family, and a higher proportion of their number have been trained in major teaching hospitals than their peers in other branches of the nursing profession[1].

It is precisely because the number of nurses working in the practice is steadily increasing that this handbook has been written. An attempt has been made to meet some of the needs of this group of nurses, who until recently often found themselves isolated in the practice with little contact with fellow practice nurses.

For the purposes of this book the term *practice nurse* will be taken to mean any nurse employed by the practice and working solely in the treatment room of the practice premises. Nevertheless, the authors hope that even those nurses who do not fall into this category may find something of interest in this book. Many of the subjects discussed may be considered controversial, and there will certainly be doctors who would not wish their nurses to undertake some of the activities outlined in later chapters. The authors would stress that they are only giving guidelines to those nurses who find themselves undertaking the activities described. The decision as to whether it is appropriate for a nurse to undertake the tasks described must be decided between the doctors and nurses in each practice.

THE DEVELOPMENT OF THE PRACTICE NURSE

In the early part of this century the general practitioner (GP) and the district nurse went very much their separate ways. Indeed, there was often distrust and hostility, especially from the doctors who disliked bureaucracy and were suspicious of the local health authorities who employed these nurses. This distrust was often mirrored by the local medical officers of health who actively discouraged the development of links between the general practitioner and the nurses.

The first glimmer of cooperation came when the far-sighted Dawson Report (1920) recommended the development of primary and secondary care by establishing health centres, where doctors and nurses could work together for the benefit of their patients. However, it was the mid-1950s before the first real collaboration occurred and experiments with the practice attachment of nurses began. In fact, the first personnel to be attached were health visitors; it was the early 1960s before district nurses began to be attached to practices on an experimental basis.

The Health Services and Public Health Act (1968) gave the seal of approval for district nurses to extend their work to seeing patients in clinics, health centres and GP premises, as well as in their own homes. It also legitimised the attachment of nurses to practices rather than on a geographical basis. When GPs became used to having nurses working with them in the practice they began to explore other ways in which they might also be employed; it was from this point that the practice nurse first came into her own.

Practice nurses began to be employed by doctors in the early 1970s when it became apparent that the district nurses (community nurses) were unable to spend a large proportion of their day on the premises doing the injections and dressing which the doctors were asking them to do. At the same time it also became clear that there were major differences in opinion between GPs and the local authority nursing hierarchy as to the role of the nurses working in the community. Many GPs were finding out that when the community nurses were working on the premises their activities were being restricted by their nursing superiors. The solution to this was for doctors to employ their own nurses, which is what an increasing number of practices did. This was paralleled at that time by the improvement of practice premises brought about by the encouraging changes of the 'GPs' Charter' of the mid-1960s, after which costs for staff and premises for family doctors were much more realistically reimbursed.

It was very difficult to determine how many doctors were employing their own nurses. Until recently, there was no specific reimbursement of practice nurse salaries and on Family Practitioner Committee returns these staff were often classified as secretaries or receptionists. However, figures now suggest that there are well over 5000 practice nurses employed throughout the country, and that this number is steadily increasing with a higher proportion in the south.

THE NURSE PRACTITIONER

The term *nurse practitioner* originates in the USA and has its counterpart in many other countries, particularly 'third world' ones. It is an attempt to meet the medical and nursing needs of the community in areas where there is little trained medical help. The nurse practitioners in the USA are particularly valuable in rural communities which have difficulty in attracting a qualified doctor to meet their needs.

Nurse practitioners in the USA undergo extra training for two years over and above that of the accredited nurse and there are not many courses where this training can take place. Extra items in the curriculum include information about diseases and the ability to prescribe a limited number of drugs. Although they normally work under the supervision of a doctor, who may be many miles away, the degree of autonomy which these nurse practitioners have is striking, and there is no doubt that they serve a valuable role in the community in which they live. Access to limited medical care is preferable to no care at all!

In the UK there has been strong resistance by the medical profession to the development of the nurse practitioner. Anxieties have been expressed about taking over the GPs' role and the profession is far from decided as to whether they wish this development to occur. Nevertheless, some advances have been made in this field and the first nurse practitioner in the UK (whose basic training was as a health visitor) took up her post in Birmingham in 1983. As yet, she is unable to prescribe drugs, which is still a jealously guarded province of the medical profession.[2]

FUTURE DEVELOPMENTS

Many developments of the past decade have ensured that the practice nurse is here to stay. These developments include:

1   The rising numbers of nurses taking this responsibility.
2   The increasing number of general practice premises with their own treatment room.
3   A change in attitude on the part of doctors who are beginning to see nurses in a partnership relationship rather than a subservient one.
4   The impact of vocational training for general practice. Young doctors, who have been trained in practices with a nurse, have become aware of her value to the work of the practice.

The time has come for the nursing and medical professions to work together to define the role of this professional. She has evolved under the pressure of changes in the pattern of workload in general practice, and through the frustration of women who felt, after having their family, that they had a great deal to offer to patients but did not want to return to the traditional hospital role. Because the development of the practice nurse has been somewhat haphazard, the definition of her role and responsibility in the practice has been slow. The defining of a role implies training for that role and the legal implications as a professional which go with it.

Since the publication of *The Training Needs of Practice Nurses* by a joint working party of the RCM, the RCGP and the BMA in 1984[3], professional development has progressed rapidly. National conferences and training programmes have been established and these developments will be discussed further in Chapter 14.

REFERENCES

1   Reedy B.L., Metcalfe A.V., de Roumaine M. and Newell D.J. (1980) The social and occupational characteristics of attached and employed nurses in general practice. *Journal of the Royal College of General Practitioners*, **30**, 477–482.
2   Stilwell B. (1984) The nurse in practice. *Nursing Mirror*, 23 May, 17–19.
3   Royal College of Nursing (1984) *The training needs of practice nurses*.

Chapter 2

Practice Organisation

THE NATIONAL HEALTH SERVICE

In 1948 the National Health Service (NHS) was established on the basis that all members of the community should have free access to medical care irrespective of their financial state. Patients should also be freed of the crippling financial effects of long term illness or expensive operations. It seems naïve now that one of the underlying principles upon which the pattern of the workload and cost was based was that in the community there was an unresolved 'pool' of illness which had not been treated because the patients could not afford it. The assumption (now proved gravely wrong!) was that once this untreated illness was given the attention of the NHS it would rapidly be cured and that while there might be an initial increased demand for care this would decrease as the population became healthier.

In the light of experience and knowledge we know now that the actual treatable illness in the population is relatively small, compared with either the chronic conditions which cannot be cured or the problems created by environmental and personal stress, which are the underlying reasons for many consultations in general practice.

Prior to 1948, those unable to afford private medical care belonged to a 'panel' of the general practitioner (GP), and their cost was supported by various insurance schemes and beds set aside in hospital especially for 'the poor'. The early days of the National Health Service were a catalogue of disaster with neither doctors nor patients really knowing what to expect of the new system. Patients had been led to believe that everything was 'free', so inordinate and unreasonable demands were made upon the GPs, who themselves were unprepared for the organisational and practical difficulties created by the new system. The medicine which doctors had learnt in medical school seemed unrelated to the problems posed by the deluge of patients attending the surgery, and many of the difficulties experienced in those early days have coloured developments in primary care since then.

During the 1950s, things slowly began to sort themselves out and amongst the new factors influencing the situation was the establishment of the College of General Practitioners in 1953. To understand subsequent developments it is important to appreciate the role of the two major bodies influencing GP opinion since that time.

The British Medical Association (BMA) through its General Medical Services Committee (GMSC) has always been responsible for the political aspects of general practice. This includes terms of service and remuneration. The College of General Practitioners (to become the Royal College in 1966) was more concerned with the educational aspects of practice, e.g. how doctors could best train themselves for the job of general practice, and how to organise their practices to provide efficient and effective primary care. The effects of these two bodies on government policies brought about in 1966 the so-called 'GPs' Charter', which radically altered the way in which GPs were paid and gave them incentives for having better premises and more staff. Prior to 1966, GPs who paid for staff or provided good premises did so entirely out of their own pocket; consequently, the doctor offering, what today would be considered normal facilities, would be financially penalised, compared with the doctor who spent the absolute minimum on his practice.

The first staff to be employed in larger numbers by GPs were reception staff and secretaries, who could perform a multitude of tasks including occasional assistance in the nursing role. Some of these staff were nurses who found more scope for their talents than just making appointments for patients. Syringes needed to be sterilised and patients prepared for minor procedures such as ear syringing and changing of dressings. It was not long before some of the more able of these nurse/receptionists were beginning to do a great deal of this routine work under the supervision of the doctor.

At this time the concept of the primary health care team was also proposed, and encouragement given for nurses and midwives to be attached to practices rather than just serve a district. The nurses concerned had undergone their hospital training, plus extra district nurse training, but their role was directed towards the nursing care of the patient at home. This has remained the traditional difference in roles between the practice nurse and her colleague in the community.

Vocational training

Even in the early days of the NHS there was some form of postgraduate training for young doctors hoping to enter practice. This took the form of a year as a trainee in an approved practice. In reality this year seldom proved to be anything other than an apprenticeship system with the doctor acting as a spare pair of hands and 'learning by doing'. This system slowly fell into disrepute and as practice vacancies as a principal became more readily available so fewer young doctors undertook a voluntary trainee year.

Matters changed in 1973 when postgraduate training for general practice was introduced on a more formal basis; this culminated in 1981 with the Vocational Training Act. It is now impossible to become a principal in general practice without three years specific postgraduate training which includes one year as a trainee in an approved practice.

General practice has come full circle in just over thirty years, from the doldrums of the early NHS when GPs were considered inferior to hospital consultants, to the present situation where a high proportion of medical students are opting for general practice as a career and taking the necessary steps to train for it.

The similarities between the development and recognition of general practice as a speciality in its own right have been compared with the difficulties facing practice nurses within their profession today.[1]

District nurse training

The aforementioned events in the medical profession have been parallelled by similar ones on the nursing side. As far back as 1889, Queen Victoria granted a Charter for the establishment of Queen Victoria's Jubilee Institute for Nurses. This was the basis of district nursing.

Within two years, training standards had been imposed upon those who wished to come under the aegis of the Queen's Institute. The first principle was to recognise the training standards, which were maintained by inspection, and the second was non-interference in a patient's religious opinion! If the nurses wished to have their names placed on the Queen's Roll they must have had at least one year's training at an approved hospital, followed by district training of not less than six months, including maternity nursing.

In 1902 the Midwives' Act was passed leading to the establishment of the Central Midwives board, giving midwives their own special recognition. In 1907, school nursing was developed, and the district nurse's role continued to widen following the First World War and the social changes occurring at that time.

The development of the home nursing services in the UK became so well-known that many other countries such as Canada, Holland, Sweden and Australia based their own community nursing services on the principles that they saw working so well in this country.

Until 1948, and the start of the National Health Service, the district nursing service was run on finance obtained entirely from voluntary sources. Local authorities took over the running of the district nursing services and in 1955 further aspects of training were debated in *Report of the Working Party on the Training of District Nurses*. In 1976 the Panel of Assessors' report, *The Education and Training of District Nurses*, was published and the official recommendation was for a six months training period plus three months supervised experience.

Health visitor training

The district nurses and midwives slowly developed their roles to the point where today there is a specific period of statutory training for both specialities and district nurses, *per se*, are no longer midwives. The same happened with health visitors.

One of the major roles of the nurse in the community has always been to educate the patients with whom she is in contact. Early health visiting activities (such as health education and preventive care) were combined in the same person, as the other nursing and midwifery roles, until the speciality of health visiting was formalised.

Today health visitors must have the RGN (SRN) qualification and at least three months midwifery experience before they are eligible to enter a specific health visitors training course. This is usually a one year course in a Polytechnic College of Further Education which includes three months of supervised training in the community. Unlike other nursing colleagues she has more statutory responsibilities within the community, e.g. the care of children under five, plus the caseload which will come from the practice within which she works.

Practice nurse training

This has been left until last in the training list, not because it is unimportant but because, as yet, there is no formal training.

The majority of those nurses undertaking practice nurse work divorced from any community nurse appointment or responsibility have tended to learn their work on a 'sink or swim' basis! Many doctors who have employed practice nurses have taken great care to train them adequately for the responsibilities which they undertake, but there are as many other practices where the nurse is really left to her own devices. The stress and dissatisfaction of this situation was reflected in the letters and enquiries made to the practice nurse subgroup of the Royal College of Nursing in the early 1980s as practice nurse numbers began to rise rapidly without a parallel development in their training facilities.

The number of nurses being employed in practices without adequate training has given rise to anxiety amongst all the professional bodies concerned, including the Royal College of Nursing and the Royal College of General Practitioners. A working party report composed by representatives of the nursing and medical professions was published in 1984 and has been responsible for many of the initiatives which have taken place since then and are discussed in Chapter 14.

The Family Practitioner Committee

The Family Practitioner Committees (FPCs) were set up as part of the organisation of the NHS to administer the remuneration and service commitments of general practitioners. In most cases they do this admirably. The actual committee, which advises the administrators, is made up of a mixture of representatives from doctors, patients, local organisations and the FPC administrators.

General practitioners are paid in a complicated way but their main sources of income within the NHS arise from:

1　A basic practice allowance paid to all general practitioners.
2　Extra supplementary allowances such as one for seniority or being a trainer.
3　Item of services fees for a wide variety of activities.
4　Dispensing fees in those rural practices which dispense.
　　In addition they get considerable financial help with:
　　(a)　Employing staff (up to a maximum of two per doctor).
　　(b)　Rent and rates for surgery premises.
　　(c)　Attending approved postgraduate refresher courses.

It is the responsibility of the FPC to record the various services which individual doctors offer and pay them quarterly for these services. A DHSS book entitled *Statement of Fees and Allowances* is given to all general practitioners and is affectionately known as 'The Red Book' because of its colour (DHSS Welsh Office 1974). This book is updated as regulations change and should be available for consultation in all practices.

PREMISES

There was a great deal of health centre development from the mid-1960s to mid-1970s as a result of government encouragement, but it has slowed down considerably since then and many doctors are now building their own premises or extending existing ones. The main reasons for increasing the size of premises have been:

1   An increase in group size with more doctors working together.
2   The addition of a treatment room.
3   Rooms for other members of the primary health care team.

A health centre is a building owned by the health authority as opposed to premises owned by the doctors. Having said that the reason why some health centres have had bad reputations is because they tend to be larger and so require more organisation to work efficiently. It is just as possible for harmonious or unhappy working conditions in either.

From the nurses' point of view there is little difference between working in a health centre or purpose-built privately-owned premises, provided both are well-designed and the practices well-organised. These aspects are considered later in this chapter.

THE NURSE IN PRACTICE

Personal care of patients and good communication between members of the primary health care team is something which has to be worked at by everyone. To this end, knowledge of fundamental management principles, the role of other members of the team and knowledge about treatment room design is essential for the practice nurse.

Management principles

There are a number of management principles which need to be applied whenever a group of people are working together, trying to run a business. The practice nurse's role involves coordinating various activities within the practice which requires an awareness and application of the relevant principles.

Responsibility for decisions

The nurse will take many decisions about the management of patients including matters such as when to see the patient again for another dressing, whether to refer a patient back to the doctor or, in the absence of other medical staff in the building, the immediate management of an emergency call which has just been received. These are just a few examples of the many responsibilities which the nurse will have. It is important that she is confident when making a decision based on her training and experience, and that the decisions themselves are supported by other members of the team, especially the doctors.

When making decisions, each team member must know the limits of his or her expertise and responsibility; the nurse must discuss these limits with the doctors or relevant team member so that the decision-making process may be clarified. Many of these discussions will take place informally on a person-to-person basis, but it is also vital to have regular meetings of the practice team.

Meetings

The more that people working together meet, informally and formally, the better they will know each other and the greater awareness there will be of each other's roles. The partners in the practice should meet regularly, at least once a month on a formal basis, to discuss practice matters and make management decisions about the running of the practice.

In addition, they should have regular meetings with the other staff to discuss problems which have arisen and also to explain future practice policy decisions. There is nothing more insidious to the sustaining of morale than decisions coming from 'on high' with no explanation, or the constant attempt by some members of the team to avoid responsibility for their actions. For a team to work closely together they need to meet frequently so that misunderstandings can be avoided or dealt with before they get out of proportion.

Rules

Part of the responsibility for decisions concerns the making of rules. All groups need guidelines—that is what rules are in this context; e.g. all staff will have the rule that matters concerning patients are not discussed outside the practice. Similarly, the practice nurse may have a rule that children who are not 100% fit do not have their routine immunisation injections. These rules have to be discussed in order for all members of staff to understand their responsibilities.

Delegation

An important principle of management is that team members should be used at a level commensurate with their ability and training. It is an inefficient use of a nurse's time for her to file patients' notes. Equally, many tasks undertaken by a doctor, such as ear syringing, are part of basic nursing training. The practice nurse will find many tasks delegated to her in this way; some of these will clearly be nursing tasks but others will depend on practice policy (e.g. a child with earache may be referred to the nurse by the receptionist if the doctors are all fully booked or occupied when the patient turns up in the surgery. The nurse may be trained to look at ear drums and distinguish the signs of otitis media and otitis externa. She may be confident and competent to do this and the doctors she works with may be happy for her to undertake this responsibility. However, if she is in doubt or the patient is obviously not satisfied, then it is the nurse's responsibility to speak to the doctor about the patient). The ultimate decision about what happens to the patient is the GP's under the terms of service which he or she has with the FPC. There will be many doctors who would consider that a child with earache should be seen by them and not referred to a nurse at all.

The fact that this situation has been discussed is not to imply that the authors approve or disapprove of this action, but only to look at the 'grey' areas in the boundaries between the role of the doctor and the nurse. In our experience most of the problems and difficulties which practice nurses have lie there, and they must be discussed fully between the professional people concerned so that responsibility is clearly defined.

The nurse herself may delegate work to either a less qualified assistant, or to a secretarial member of staff if clerical work needs to be done. Again it is a waste of a nurse's training to spend a lot of time on clerical activities if patients require nursing attention but it will be her responsibility to see that relevant patient data is entered in the records.

Sharing information and feedback

Much of this section has already been covered or implied in the section on meetings. Like hospital team work, it is vital when a group of people work together in a practice that necessary information is shared so that patients benefit maximally when their care involves several people. Part of this information sharing lies in the keeping of good records, but some will be verbal, as will matters relating to other aspects of organisation in the practice.

Feedback involves the giving of information about the consequences of action already taken. This may be in the form of the doctor telling the nurse what happened later to a patient whom she previously treated. It also has wider implications for the practice in terms of management. This relates to such matters as workload and appointment systems. If sufficient patients complain that they cannot get appointments or that they have to wait a long time to be seen then this feedback needs to be acted upon.

These are the major principles of management as they affect the practice nurse. Much of what has been said would seem to be commonsense. In a small one-or-two-doctor practice with a handful of staff a great deal of communication will take place informally because the staff are in frequent contact. However, nurses may find themselves working in larger premises with many staff; then it becomes more important to have matters formalised so that misunderstandings and mismanagement do not occur.

THE PRACTICE TEAM

When working together each member of the practice team must know and understand the background training, the roles and the responsibilities of the others. Some of the more important aspects of the training and responsibilities of various personnel with whom the nurse will work are outlined.

The practice manager

Larger practices require someone to take over the responsibility of organising the day-to-day activities. The person appointed as practice manager may be a senior secretary/receptionist who has 'grown up' through the system and become manager almost by default. This can be a positive advantage as that person will know the other staff well, their various needs and the peculiarities of the practice from long acquaintance with them.

A new breed of practice manager is now appearing with more specific managerial training. These personnel are often men and are found in the larger health centres or group practices. Their background is frequently the Services or another administrative post within the NHS. However the manager is appointed the responsibilities remain much the same. These include:

1 Day-to-day organisation of the practice.
2 Appointment of staff and staff contracts.
3 Liaison with the practice accountant and some book-keeping.
4 Liaison with all members of the practice team and responsibility for organising regular practice meetings.
5 Ordering of supplies.
6 Secretarial and reception duties.

There is a formal organisation to which managers can belong called the Organisation of Health Centre Administrators and Practice Managers. This does arrange some training courses and symposia, and other management courses are occasionally run by polytechnic colleges or organisations such as the local faculty of the Royal College of General Practitioners.

Receptionist/secretary

A practice must have pleasant, willing reception staff who give a good impression to patients and other visitors. The most important characteristics for these staff are a pleasant personality and the ability to stay calm under conflicting demands from many directions simultaneously—doctors, patients and telephones.

The Association of Medical Secretaries (AMSPAR) have a one- or two-year training course available at some polytechnic colleges. This type of course, however, may be more orientated towards the full-time hospital secretary rather than the part-time receptionist who has taken up a job after having had a family or moving from some other type of work. Many reception staff have to train in service and are expected to pick up the skills as they gain more experience.

Secretarial qualifications are gained through secretarial schools. It is helpful to have at least one of the staff with these skills to write referral letters and other practice correspondence although she will need a medical dictionary to help with terminology.

The reception staff themselves are responsible for:

1 Running an efficient appointment system.
2 Taking messages by telephone.
3 Preparing patient records for the next surgery and filing them afterwards.
4 Operating various practice systems such as repeat prescribing or recall systems.
5 Miscellaneous tasks not covered by anyone else.

The community nurse

It is most important that the practice nurse and the various members of the community nursing team get on well together and understand each other's roles. In some areas the community nurse may also work for some part of the day in the treatment room and if a practice nurse is also employed by the practice, difficulties in role perception can arise. It is more common though in those practices who employ practice nurses for the community nurse to only work outside the practice premises.

The main responsibility of the community nurse is to provide nursing services to those patients for whom she or he is responsible in the community. Many of these nurses are based at practices or health centres where everybody gets to know each other, but in some areas the community nurses will be working on an area basis and not specifically for one practice. The advantage to the nursing hierarchy of this system is that they are more easily able to organise the available manpower, but the disadvantage is that no person is clearly identified with whom a practice can discuss patient problems.

The community nurses have their own nursing hierarchy of command, in the District Community Nursing services, and are ultimately responsible to their superiors there. This can create some problems for them if the doctors see their role as different from that seen by their nursing officers (e.g. misunderstanding and argument has occurred when community nurses have been asked to immunise patients or take blood samples when their superiors have not seen this as an appropriate task for them).

Most of the nursing services which they perform are familiar to practice nurses as they both have a common hospital training. While practice nurses are by definition RGN (Registered General) (see Chapter 1) the community nursing team works similarly to the ward team concept with mixed skills and grades. The team leader must be a district nurse and the other members will be a mixture of RGN, EN(G) and auxilliaries.

In order to qualify as a district nurse the RGN must have at least two years of post basic training in hospital, followed by a one year course at a university or polytechnic college. Much of the time is spent in conjunction with a health visitors' course.

The community midwife

Most practices have a community midwife attached to them or attending for various antenatal sessions. She must be a State Certified Midwife and is responsible for organising the antenatal and postnatal care in the practice. If the sessions are busy she may welcome the help of the practice nurse in the routine management of the patients (see Chapter 11).

The midwife will attend the confinement if it is at home or in a GP hospital unit and will then attend the mother and baby daily until the tenth day after delivery, in the majority of cases. In exceptional circumstances, she may have to attend for a little longer than ten days. If the patient is confined in hospital but discharged before the tenth day then she is responsible for daily care from the time the patient returns home until the tenth day. She is also responsible for running relaxation classes and parentcraft classes, perhaps with the help of the health visitor.

The health visitor

The recognised case load for a health visitor is one visitor to 4000 patients, so some practices will have one or more attached health visitors but others will share her skills if the patient numbers in the practice are too few or the full complement of health visitors is not employed.

The health visitor has to be a RGN nurse, have a minimum of three months' midwifery training (but not necessarily be a State Registered Midwife) and then have attended a one-year health visitors' course held at certain colleges of further education. She has statutory responsibilities, particularly for children, and is responsible for running developmental clinics and all aspects of health care and screening in the community.

Their remit is so wide that the majority find themselves very busy just keeping up with the case load produced by clinics, and day-to-day problems arising in the practice and referred to them by the GP or other members of the team. Sometimes a health visitor with specific responsibility for the elderly in the area will be appointed, and is of particular value in parts of the country where there is a high geriatric component due to patients retiring there (e.g. seaside resorts on the south coast).

The health visitor is an important professional in her own right with more organisational than nursing responsibilities but the practice nurse will find it useful to liaise closely with her, particularly where the 'under five' patients in the practice are concerned.

Social worker

Prior to the reorganisation of the NHS in 1974 and the Seebohm Report on the role of the social worker, these members of the primary health care team were often nurses with a special interest (e.g. psychiatry). They took extra training to become social workers in a special field such as psychiatric social workers or child care officers. However, under the new regulations, all social workers had to have a common basic training and be able to cope with all aspects of social work rather than just one. The other result of reorganisation was that experienced social workers suddenly found themselves being promoted into administrative posts leaving few experienced workers in the community. For these and other reasons, relationships between the rest of the primary health care team and social workers has not been as close or efficient as it might have been. Far fewer practices have a social worker specifically attached, compared with the other professionals of the primary health care team, and this also hinders efficient communication between the members.

Social workers are responsible for a wide number of problem areas, including welfare benefits, housing and deprived families, as well as being involved in such activities as counselling or organising community care. Within the practice team they are most likely to liaise with the GP or health visitor, but the practice nurse should know when a particular problem might be helped by referral to a social worker.

THE PRACTICE WORKLOAD

It is inevitable that everyone in the practice thinks that he or she is working very hard and that the constant battle of supply and demand will never be won. There are, however, certain guiding principles to consider when looking at the practice workload and the ways in which patients are seen.

Appointment system

Many practices now have appointment systems, but if the rules are applied too rigidly, then patient dissatisfaction occurs because the waiting time for an appointment may be quite inappropriate.

Doctors should give specific instructions about the number of patients whom they wish to see per hour. It is their responsibility to see that they make themselves available for a realistic number of hours compared with the size of the practice list. There is no point in saying that he or she will see ten patients an hour, starting at 9.00 a.m., and then persistently arrive at 9.30 a.m. and consult at a rate of six patients an hour. This type of behaviour causes congestion in the waiting room, anger in the patients and frustration in the receptionists! It also means that patients may get directed to the practice nurse inappropriately because of pressure upon the receptionist to fit them in somewhere. The practice nurse should have an appointment book too. The staff should record what procedure the appointment is for (e.g. removal of a wart, dressing an ulcer or taking a blood sample). It is important to know approximately how long the nursing procedures will take if the system is to function efficiently. It will be the responsibility of the practice nurse to tell the staff this information so that allowance can be made for the time-consuming activities. It is a good idea to book non-urgent activities such as ECGs or varicose ulcer dressings in the slack periods of the day, away from the time when surgeries are being run and the doctors may require the practice nurse's services for other work.

When patients regularly have to spend a long time in the waiting room before being seen by the nurse or the doctor then the appointment system should be reconsidered. Urgent cases must be seen the same day as the request. When it appears that patients are having to wait several days for an appointment then this should also be considered. Some form of feedback should be built into the system, so that those operating it are aware of snags and blocks before they become too insurmountable.

All practices have occasions when the demands of the population seem overwhelming. This may be due to an influenza epidemic or to the social problems of a new town; whatever the cause, there is always a way of reorganising things so that life becomes more tolerable again. This is where the principles of management, such as delegation, are so important.

In addition to these principles, a well-designed treatment room will help considerably to lighten the load of the practice nurse.

Treatment room design

During the rapid development of health centre premises in the decade 1965–75, many lessons were learnt about the best way to design buildings for primary care. Unfortunately, not all these lessons were heeded and the same mistakes were made time and time again. There is now a considerable volume of literature about the design of premises, but the main features to insist upon are that:

1   The room should be light, airy and not too 'clinical'.
2   There must be ample cupboard space and worktops. Remember that equipment, dressings, sample bottles and forms of one sort or another have all to be stored in the treatment room.
3   There should be a hatch access to a toilet for the collecting of urine samples.
4   There should be several work areas, preferably with their own couches, so that a number of patients can be accommodated simultaneously. This is particularly important if more than one nurse at a time is going to work in the room.
5   A separate room with a couch is available, which can be used for isolating infectious cases or for use as a recovery room.
6   If minor operations are to be performed there must be ample room for these activities and suitable sterilising equipment available.
7   The treatment room should be adjacent to the GP consulting suites so that easy communication between the two is possible.
8   Where possible, incorporate a separate waiting area for the treatment room; this prevents confusion between those patients waiting for the doctor and those waiting for the nurse.
9   There are adequate electrical power points. With the future in mind, it might be worth considering the installation of a

computer point for multi-user systems in new premises. Smaller premises using a computer would probably have the desk top stand alone variety and the need for outlets would not then apply.

10 Separate office space is valuable where confidential interviews and counselling can take place and all the paperwork can be completed.

Some of the design guidelines mentioned might seem obvious to a nurse familiar with working in a treatment room. However, it is surprising how often simple design faults are made (e.g. the siting of lights). When new premises are planned, it is important that the practice nurse is involved, and has a say in the design of her treatment room. Although the architect will have specific ideas, the practice nurse must comment on these if they seem inappropriate. Many beautiful buildings have been designed which are nice to look at but awful to work in! A good architect will seek opinions because only the person who has to perform the tasks in a room designed for certain functions will have a clear idea of the best way to meet those needs.

Probably the most effective way of clarifying your own thoughts on the matter are to visit, preferably with your doctors, other practices who have recently built premises. Talk to the staff and get their opinions, particularly on the faults or innovative ideas, and look critically at the rooms which you will use to see whether you would feel comfortable working there. Whatever the answer, try and analyse why the design is good or bad, then use this information in your own plans.

Practice organisation is a difficult but important area of general practice. The fundamental message is that all members of the team should be involved in the practice and ensure that their professional opinions are both wanted and useful.

REFERENCES

1 Bolden K.J. and Bolden S. (1986) Is history repeating itself? *British Medical Journal*, 293, 19–20.

Chapter 3

Record Systems

A good record system is vital for any form of patient management to function efficiently. This is true more so now that the team concept of care is accepted, and a number of professionals may all be involved with an individual patient. Gone are the days of the solo general practitioner (GP), who knew his patients individually and tried to keep all the relevant information about them in his head, without committing anything to paper.

In vocational training practices, the standard of records is expected to be high, so that the GP trainee can have all the information about a patient available to him or her during the consultation. The increasing emphasis on preventive care in the community means that record systems also have to include other data, such as immunisation or cervical smears, and not just the patients' medical history. In addition retrieval methods have to be built into the system so that patients can be recalled for various repeat activities (e.g. cervical smears every five years on women over 35 years of age). Finally, the ability to identify patients suffering from particular diseases, such as diabetes or hypertension, is of value when organising clinics for the routine management of these cases or for training purposes in teaching practices.

Any system of record keeping must incorporate these features if it is to meet the challenge of modern general practice. The practice nurse should be a major contributor to the information contained within this system and will probably be responsible for many of the preventive care aspects of it. To this end she must, therefore, understand the way in which record systems are set up and the correct use of the information recorded.

PURPOSE OF A RECORD

The purpose of a record is:

1   To record all relevant medical information about a patient.

2   To include other important aspects, such as the family and social history of the patient.
3   To enable preventive care to be offered to appropriate patients.
4   To facilitate the management of patients with chronic illness.
5   To enable all members of the primary health care team to work together to the benefit of the patient.
6   To act as a focus for the education of trainee GPs or other members of the primary health care team in training.
7   To enable data to be extracted for practice audit performance review and research purposes.

THE MEDICAL RECORD ENVELOPE

The medical record envelope (MRE) is familiar to all personnel working in general practice as it has been the main source of written information about the patient since 1911. It was originally known as the 'Lloyd George' envelope as it was introduced during the time when Lloyd George was Prime Minister. The fact that it has been around for so long says something for its durability but also explains why in the 1980s its size may seem somewhat inadequate for today's needs! However, it is still in common usage and is capable of being adapted to meet most of the purposes outlined although it is only 17.5 × 12.5 cm.

Contents

The continuation cards in the record should be in chronological order and tagged together. Letters should be trimmed to fit the envelope easily and all irrelevant material destroyed by the doctor. Letters should also be filed in chronological order and fastened together, preferably by treasury tags rather than clips or staples, as this allows easier access to the information. Data in the records should be written legibly (or typed) and it is helpful to outline, in a box, any major diagnosis or events so that they stand out clearly.

Besides this simple and very basic record which is now the absolute minimum expected in training practices, there are a number of insert cards which can be obtained to expand the information available.

Summary card

The summary card (pink or blue) is used to summarise all the important information about the patient. It is time-consuming to keep these cards updated as new information becomes available, but this must be done if they are to be of practical use. A member of the secretarial staff should be responsible for this.

Inclusion of a summary record card is becoming a training requirement in many parts of the country.

Repeat prescription or treatment card

The way in which repeat prescriptions are kept under control is more the responsibility of the office staff and details will not be given of the various methods available. However, an insert card with details of present and recurrent treatment is of value to the nurse since she may be asked to obtain repeat presciptions for the patient. All requests *must* be entered in the record so that it is known when the patient last had the item, and, because it is not desirable for any patient to go on indefinitely having repeat prescriptions, an occasional review by the doctor should be organised.

Contraceptive record card

Some practitioners use a contraceptive record card so that routine items (e.g. blood pressure check, cervical smears or contraceptive claim forms (FP1001/2)) can be recorded in such a way that it is obvious if something has been forgotten. There are a number of other examples of special record cards such as this, and they have a limited place which is usually dictated by the enthusiasm of the practice for completing them and the size of the record envelope in accommodating them.

Obstetric record card

Antenatal patients carry an obstetric record card to the various clinics which they attend during pregnancy. This enables medical staff to be aware of the information recorded at the previous visits. At the postnatal examination, the record card should be inserted in the medical records envelope, so that it is available for reference in future pregnancies if required.

Developmental assessment chart for children under five years of age

Developmental assessment clinics used to be organised by the health authority but many practices now arrange their own. Two types of record are required, one is a list of items to be checked at various ages and the other is a percentile chart for height and weight so that the child can be assessed in regard to others of his or her own age.

It is possible to combine this type of record with the preventive care record so that data from all sources is recorded in one place. This will obviously be preferable if the number of cards kept in the MRE continues to expand.

OTHER SYSTEMS

A4 records

Mention has already been made of the small size of the 'Lloyd George' envelope. Some doctors have become impatient with the limitations imposed upon them by this size and, since the early 1970s, a number of practices have gone over to A4 (297 × 210 cm) records, which is the standard size for hospital notes. All staff who have access to the records will find advantages and disadvantages in this system.

This system has three advantages.

1 The record is larger and can open out with all the letters flat and easily read.
2 There is more space to record information.
3 It can incorporate extra records, such as summary cards, without the congestion caused in the small envelopes.

There are also three disadvantages.

1 With the exception of Scotland and certain experiments financed separately in England, most practices will have to pay the cost of transferring their records to an A4 system.
2 The records are much larger and, therefore, require more storage space in the office.
3 The increase in size, and the effort of transferring to the system, may induce a complacency in the doctors that their records are now satisfactory. This is not true and just as much effort is required to keep them legible and updated as with the simpler system.

The computer

Computerised record systems in practice are now becoming a reality and many doctors are beginning to experiment with them. It will be some time yet before the systems are adapted sufficiently for the needs of general practice, and a considerable amount of time before their use is widespread. However, their introduction will ease the nurse's role in using recall systems while probably increasing the number of activities available to her.

Microcomputer systems, either stand alone (single) systems or multi-user ones, are becoming widely available and will eventually replace all the card systems described in this chapter. The scope is vast and practices who invest in a computer system wonder how they managed without one!

Staff should not regard their introduction as a threat or refuse to become involved but regard them as an essential practice tool in the same way as any other piece of equipment which is used routinely.

Age/sex register

Mention will be made frequently in this book about the importance of *preventive care* and the role of the practice nurse in this activity, but no practice can begin to offer methodical and comprehensive preventive care to the patients unless an age/sex register is in operation to do this. Basically this is a register of all the patients in the practice divided into groups by age and sex. There are two types of manual register available; a book and a card file.

The book system

A looseleaf book may be used with each page representing a year (e.g. 1890, 1920 or 1945). All patients in the practice are recorded in the book under the year of their birth and categorised according to sex (e.g. if all female patients born in 1979 are required for rubella immunisation, then the page or pages relevant to this year would be consulted and the patients sent for). The disadvantage of this system is that only the patient's name can be recorded, and as patients leave the practice they will be crossed out, so the pages soon look untidy.

The card system

The Royal College of General Practitioners has produced a set of pink or blue cards to organise an age/sex register. Each patient has a card on which there is space for other items of information to be recorded, where appropriate, and then the cards are stored in a box file by year. This system is simple, inexpensive and effective and has room for other details about the patient too.

Recall systems

Part of preventive care activities include having a method of recalling patients after certain specified periods of time (e.g. five-yearly) for a cervical smear. A simple card system for this can be introduced along the lines of the age/sex card register. Each patient has a card that is filed by the year and month when the patient is to be recalled. As each time interval comes up the patients on the cards concerned are sent for by the practice secretary. A similar system can be used for many different types of recall but normally it is not possible to operate more than about six recall systems of this sort manually. It is particularly in this area of record keeping that computers will prove of great value.

The practice nurse will have to be familiar with the various recall systems available and the criteria for recall, since she will have the responsibility for arranging the preventive care activities involved whether it be giving a baby an immunisation or checking the blood pressure of a middle-aged man.

Disease register

An increasing interest is being shown by GPs in identifying certain disease groups amongst their patients (e.g. diabetes or hypertension). A colour code tagging system was adopted by the Royal College of General Practitioners and has now become universally accepted. The code is:

Brown — diabetes
Yellow — epilepsy
Blue — hypertension
Red — sensitivity to drugs
Purple — cancer
Green — tuberculosis (TB)
Black — attempted suicide

The front of the patient's notes can have a colour tag on it to remind the doctor of the condition at the time of the consultation. Other colour codes and systems are now being used as well and may prove confusing to the staff. However, more importantly, the age/sex cards can be colour tagged over the edge of the card uppermost in the file so that just by looking at the cards in the box file all those cards tagged with a specific colour can immediately be identified. This simple system will then give the practice a modified disease register, whereby patients suffering from six or eight major diseases can be immediately identified for preventive care, management or teaching purposes.

A much more complex system involves the use of a book (called an E book) to record many more diseases than those mentioned. It is beyond the scope of this book to go into the details of this because few practices use them and the practice nurse is unlikely to be involved.

When computerisation becomes common practice, a simple indication of the patient's disease in the data system will enable a comprehensive list of patients suffering from any condition to be immediately printed out on request, and will render these simple tagging systems obsolete.

As the practice nurse's role expands, the responsibility for routine administration of the follow-up of patients with certain diseases (e.g. diabetes or hypertension) will increasingly be part of her work. Familiarity with the various records and registers is an integral part of this responsibility.

CONFIDENTIALITY

Nurses are trained to follow the same ethical code as doctors — to respect the confidence of patients and ensure that confidential information is not broadcast to those for whom it is not intended. We re-emphasise the importance of confidentiality in a world where information systems are growing and the privacy of the individual is constantly being eroded.

It has been said that the main contribution of the GP record to confidentiality was its chaos and illegibility! Now that records are becoming more structured and the information more readily accessible for medical purposes it also opens up the way for unauthorised people, such as cleaners, to have access to it. All staff working in primary care should have the importance of the principle of confidentiality impressed upon them, but non-medical personnel do not always view these matters in quite the same way as doctors and nurses. It is important that no casual gossip is carried outside about activities in the practice, and information acquired about patients should not be disclosed without the patient's permission. This restriction equally applies to information given to someone on the other end of a telephone, purporting to be a relative of the patient. In these circumstances, information which may cause the patient harm or imply to him or her that confidences have been broken must not be divulged. The ethical and confidential aspects of the work must be emphasised by the doctors or practice manager when any new member of staff joins the practice. The same principles apply to the written record. If records are left open or lying around at the end of the day then the temptation for other people to look at them will be increased. Records should certainly be filed as quickly as possible, and letters and laboratory results inserted into the record as soon as they have been read by the doctor.

Anxiety has been expressed about computers and confidentiality. This has mainly been because of the large volume of data stored upon them and the number of personnel using the computer. If the computer system is based in the practice then this is not a real problem and, indeed, is more secure than the written file because anyone with access to the information can be identified. Entry codes and passwords can be designed to limit the amount of access to the record to specific staff.

National storage of patient data is a different matter and has given legitimate cause for concern over the last few years. Medical staff must consider carefully what information is appropriate to refer centrally. This must never be done without careful consultation with all those involved.

Data Protection Act (1987)

The Data Protection Act (1987) gave patients the right to see their own medical record. If this request is made, then a number of issues may be considered:

(a) the request does not need to be acceded to immediately but has to be met within 40 days
(b) records should not contain trivial or rude comments about patients
(c) the request should usually be responded to by a counselling interview to explore why the request was made. Often patients ask because of unstated anxieties about their health which become apparent in discussion and can be dealt with
(d) does the record contain significant information, for example about the prognosis of an illness that the patient does not know? If so, what will be the consequences to the patient of finding out?

It is difficult to generalise but if a practice follows a philosophy of respect for the patient, a sharing of information and a joint responsibility for care, then problems are unlikely to arise.

Nevertheless, new ethical issues are becoming common, for example, HIV results, and the situation should be kept under constant review in the practice.

Chapter 4

Assessment and Evaluation of the Patient

When a nurse joins a practice she will need to discuss with the doctors the way in which she is going to work and what they perceive as her role in the practice. She will also have her own perceptions of the post and its responsibilities, and these should be discussed openly with the partners. A relationship based on a mutual professional respect and an awareness of the roles and responsibilities of all members of the practice team is important and will certainly speed the integration of a close and happy working relationship.

The general practitioners should already have decided between themselves what are to be the areas of responsibility for the nurse and they should discuss these areas with her to see that they all agree on the practice nurse role. Practice policy on procedures for the practice nurse should be clearly set out (e.g. policies concerning life-threatening emergencies, see Chapter 8). The exact scope and responsibility of the nurse will be governed by her previous experience and training, such as the making of management decisions and action to be taken if a doctor is not on the premises when a problem arises.

Patients will come to the practice nurse in one of four ways.

1 Referred by the doctor for some procedure or dressing.
2 Referred by the receptionist either because a doctor is not readily available or she perceives the problem to be an appropriate nursing problem (e.g. routine ear syringing or minor injuries).
3 Follow-up visit for some procedure already initiated (e.g. dressings or routine injections).
4 Self-referral by the patient who perceives the nurse as being suitable to help with their particular problem.

The assessment of the needs of the patient attending the treatment room may be very simple (e.g. the doctor may have requested a blood sample to be taken for a haemoglobin estimation). However, many patients' needs are more complex and it is only after a great deal of experience that the practice nurse may feel confident to make her own decision about the management of a particular patient. Whatever the problem some general guidelines are applicable to most situations.

General guidelines

1 Talk to the patient to help decide why he or she is seeing you and to determine through which particular referral system (*see above*) the patient arrived in the treatment room.
2 For patients referred by a doctor most activities will be straightforward, as he or she will have already assessed the situation clinically and made a management decision. However, the request from the doctor may not always be clear or it may be for an unfamiliar procedure or sample. A difficult situation may arise when a nurse is requested to carry out a procedure for which she has not been properly trained or to do a test (such as for HIV titre) where she is not sure that the patient is fully informed about the consequences of it. In every case she should remember that she has a professional and ethical responsibility to be certain that her actions are in the best interests of the patient. If in any doubt contact the doctor and discuss the problem before proceeding further.
3 Patients who are referred to the nurse by the receptionist may have been referred appropriately or not. A patient who has asked for an appointment to see the doctor and been referred for your opinion because an appointment is not readily available can be most difficult to assess. The patient may feel aggrieved not to be seeing the doctor, although most patients soon become familiar with the presence of practice nurses and feelings of distrust or irritation are usually minimal or not present at all. It is important to be pleasant and not respond in an officious or critical manner with these patients to defuse any possible aggression in these circumstances. Usually these feelings are, in any case, precipitated only by the patient's anxiety about the problem and one not related to the nurse personally.

Many patients referred in this way will have problems that can be dealt with by the nurse. However, the guiding principle must again be, if in doubt, ask for further advice from the doctor. It may be that giving the doctor details of the problem and your assessment of it will be sufficient for him or her to make a management decision based upon that information without needing to see the patient. The medico-legal implication of management decisions by nurses and doctors will be discussed again in Chapter 13, but essentially decisions without referral should only be taken in those areas clearly defined as a practice nurse's responsibility by discussion between the doctor and nurse.

4   Between one-third and one-half of the treatment room workload will be related to repeat procedures on patients who have been assessed and evaluated previously. In the case of repeated dressing for wounds or varicose ulcers, the necessary decisions to be taken are:

(a)   Is the condition progressing satisfactorily?
If not, does it need repeat referral to the doctor?
(b)   Does the present treatment need to be continued and for how long?
(c)   When should the patient attend again?

As far as repeat procedures such as a course of iron injections or other long term medication is concerned, it is important to know how long the course is intended to continue. If it is indefinitely, when is the patient to be reviewed by the doctor?

5   The patients who refer themselves to the nurse are always professionally satisfying. They have usually had previous contact with the nurse and often have established a rapport. The nurse will have to determine whether the patient's decision to ask for her advice alone is correct and, when asked for an opinion, whether it is within her professional experience or expertise. (It may be helpful to both doctors and nurses to have some of the more formal procedures written down as guidelines and an example of the way in which this might be done is shown in Appendix IX.)

Without discussing individual cases it is not possible to give further guidance about management, but it is hoped that the information contained in this book, together with experience and confidence, will enable the practice nurse to make patient management decisions safely and correctly. Until professional experience has built up in this difficult area it is well to remember that it is better to be 'safe than sorry'! The doctors should always be supportive when the practice nurse seeks advice no matter how busy they may be themselves.

Chapter 5

Nursing Procedures

General and basic nursing skills are taught during general nursing training. The aims of this chapter are to discuss nursing activities specific to general practice. These skills and procedures often vary from hospital nursing and so need specialised degrees of skill, training and responsibility.

INJECTIONS

These can be grouped in three sections:

1 Routine immunisations and vaccinations which will be discussed fully in Chapter 7.
2 Prophylactic injections for travelling abroad will also be discussed in Chapter 7.
3 Other injections, e.g. Iron (Jectofer), flupenthixol (Depixol), cyano-cobalamin (Cytamen), penicillin, myocrisin, depot steroids (Kenalog) and desensitising vaccines.

Other injections

Usually specialised injections for a patient are categorised as 'other'. The patient obtains the appropriate injection on prescription from the general practitioner. The injection can be given into the upper arm, thigh or upper outer quadrant of the buttock, according to the type of injection. The site of these specialised injections should be discussed with the doctor, and an agreed format followed for each one.

The practice nurse should always be familiar with the manufacturers advice sheet and follow any recommendations given in it. A record of the date and amount of the dose, together with the manufacturers name and batch number of the injection, should be made in the notes. The Product Liability Act (1988) made the dispenser of a drug (in this case the GP and nurse) liable for the consequences of any adverse side effects if that responsibility could not be transferred to a named manufacturer. After recording these details the nurse should arrange a recall date with the patient for the next injection where this is appropriate.

Desensitising vaccines are not commonly given in practice now as a number of deaths have occurred from severe anaphylactic reactions (Chapter 8). Full resuscitation equipment should be available if these injections are given, but even then there are risks that the patient will collapse with a secondary reaction after leaving the surgery.

DRESSINGS

The principles for dressings are the same as those taught in general nursing training. Occasionally patients are taught to re-dress simple wounds at home, although most patients prefer to attend the treatment room. The dressings which are dealt with by the practice nurse are usually referred from the doctor, from hospital (either from casualty or postoperatively), from the community nurse (if the patient becomes mobile enough to attend the surgery) or self-referred by the patient. The most common types of dressing dealt with by the practice nurse are for:

1   Venous and arterial ulcers
2   Postoperative abdominal wounds
3   Removal of sutures
4   Re-dressing injuries
5   Burns and scalds
6   Abscesses, boils and infected cysts
7   Ingrowing toenails
8   Eye dressings.

1   Venous and arterial ulcers

Dressings for varicose ulcers are usually referred to the nurse by the GP. The practice nurse then takes responsibility for the dressings and assessment of the condition. The doctor makes the decision on treatment and discusses management with the nurse, who is then responsible for the regular dressings and should always evaluate the condition of the wound, referring the matter to the doctor if the condition is not improving or if, in her opinion, the treatment needs changing or reassessing.

The specialised sterile dressings or bandages which are used are obtained on prescription for each patient. A level of stock dressings should be maintained in the treatment room. When caring for leg ulcers in the treatment room it is more satisfactory for the patient to visit the surgery no more than once a day although preferably once or twice a week.

Also consideration should be given to the condition of the patient, the home situation and any family ties and before treatment and management commences the type of ulcer must be correctly diagnosed as either arterial or venous.

Arterial ulcers

1 These usually develop between and at the tips of toes, over phalangeal heads, on heels and above the lateral malleolus.
2 It has a well demarcated edge, is deep with pale base, necrosis and absence of healthy granulation tissue. Around the ulcer the skin may be shiny and dry and the toenails thickened. The leg may become pale when elevated.
3 It is very painful—the pain is brought on by ischaemia as well as the ulcer itself.
4 There is decreased or absent arterial pulsation at the routine check points in the leg.

Venous ulcers

1 These usually develop in the gaiter area at the ankle, pre-tibial and anteromedial supramalleolar areas.
2 Venous ulcers are usually superficial with uneven edges and ruddy granulation tissue. Around the ulcer may be oedema, reddish brown discolouration and dilated tortuous superficial veins.
3 Infected venous ulcers may be painful but often patients are pain-free.

The management and treatment of arterial and venous ulcers should be approached differently. Patients with *arterial ulcers* need light bandaging to protect ischaemic tissues from further trauma and the leg should not be elevated as this will compound the ischaemic problems. The patient should avoid tight shoes, raise the head of bed, use a cradle in the bed and sheepskin support under heel to prevent further tissue damage.

Patients with *venous ulcers* need support bandaging to eliminate oedema and reduce venous hypertension. The leg should be elevated above the level of the heart and active ankle movements should be maintained to improve venous return by activating the calf pump mechanism. The patient should be encouraged to walk as much as possible. When a venous ulcer is healed elastic support hose should be worn and can be obtained on prescription.

Suggestions for methods of cleaning and dressing leg ulcers
Cleansing agents and dressings

The aim of a cleansing agent is to clean without destroying granulation tissue.

1 Saline—effective, simple, used before a covering dressing.
2 Savlodyl—gentle and effective.
3 Chlorhexidine—gentle and effective, bactericidal.
4 Eusol—often damages tissue, use with care.
5 Eusol and paraffin—paraffin encourages bacterial growth.
6 Varidase—expensive, needs to be used twice daily, excellent results on sloughing ulcers.
7 Debrisan—expensive, once or twice daily use. Excellent in ulcers with a high exudate (absorbs seven times own weight in exudate).
8 Iodosorb—expensive, changed daily, each time the dressing is changed the remaining Iodosorb should be gently washed from the ulcer surface.

Antiseptic wet dressings
These are the most suitable treatments for the infected or exudative ulcer. The skin around the ulcer can be protected with zinc oxide paste.

9 Potassium permanganate 1:10,000 dilution.
10 5% hydrogen peroxide.
11 Benoxyl 20 volume solution—three or four gauze squares cut to the size of the wound soaked in the solution and placed on ulcer, a plastic sheet cut to slightly larger size. Ideally this should be changed twice daily as the exudate irritates the surrounding skin, however once daily may suffice.

Antiseptic creams, ointments or sprays
These dressings are used for the less exudative ulcers and have the advantage of needing to be changed three or four times per week. The wound is first cleaned with sterile normal saline.

12 Flamazine cream (silver sulphadiazine).
13 Disadine—dry powder spray containing 0.5% povidone iodine.

Impregnated tulle dressings
14 Jelonet—plain paraffin tulle dressing.
15 Bactigras—paraffin tulle impregnated with 0.5% chlorhexidine acetate.
16 Fucidin intertulle—2% sodium fucidate.
17 Sofra tulle—1% framycetin sulphate.
18 Honey tulle—honey and cod liver oil.

Paste bandages

These are based on a zinc paste bandage, are useful when eczema is extensive and can be used with all types of ulcers even exudative ones. The advantage of these bandages is that they need changing no more than once per week.

19 Viscopaste—plain.
20 Ichthopaste, Ichthaband—with ichthamol.
21 Quinaband—with calamine.

Other measures

22 Opsite—film seal dressing. epithilealisation can be observed.
23 Granuflex—is a flexible hydroactive dressing, keeps the ulcer moist which aids migration of epidermal cells.
24 Silastic foam.

Oral treatments

25 Diuretic—may be prescribed to reduce peripheral oedema.
26 Antibiotic—for cellulitis or lymphangitis.
27 Stromba—aids build up of cells and granulating tissue, of doubtful value.
28 Vitamins or iron—some patients have low iron or folate levels and may need these supplements.

Surgical procedures

29 Grafts—are occasionally performed.

Important factors when dealing with ulcers

1 Reassess with the doctor at regular intervals.
2 Measure for size to assess progress or deterioration.
3 Know when to change the treatment.
4 Know the suitable dressings available.
5 Do not continue with same treatment indefinitely, especially if matters are not improving.

2 Postoperative abdominal wounds

Postoperative abdominal wounds which require dressings are usually referred from hospital wards, outpatient or hospital casualty departments. Often patients are discharged from hospital casualty departments and from hospital requiring regular changes of dressings. The practice nurse will have a communication from the hospital stating the type of dressing to be undertaken. She is then responsible for the routine treatment. Once again the sterile specialised dressings are obtained by prescription from the general practitioner.

3   Removal of sutures or clips

Patients who need sutures or clips removed may be referred from hospital or after surgery in the treatment room. The practice nurse is responsible for making the decision when the sutures or clips are ready for removal (usually about a week after insertion) and for re-dressing and observing the wound afterwards.

4   Re-dressing injuries

Most patients with injuries are referred either by self or by GP. The practice nurse is competent to assess the severity of the wound and will either refer to the doctor or decide the management herself. For minor cuts, abrasions, bruises or sprains the nurse can be responsible for cleaning, evaluating and advising, and when necessary applying the appropriate treatment.

If, after evaluation, the nurse considers the injury is severe the patient must be referred to the doctor. These injuries would include those needing suturing, severe abrasions or injuries possibly requiring an X-ray. In all instances the patient's current state of vaccination against tetanus should be checked and if necessary a course commenced.

If the injury is the result of an accident or incident where litigation might be involved (e.g. a road accident) then the doctor should see the patient, even if the injury is trivial, and record the details in case a report has to be written later.

The detailed management of more severe orthopaedic injuries can be found elsewhere[1].

5   Burns and scalds

When a patient arrives in the treatment room with a burn or scald, first aid treatment has usually been administered. Severe burns or scalds must always be referred to the doctor but minor burns can be managed by the practice nurse.

For burns or scalds of hands and fingers, cream silver sulphadiazine 1% (Flamazine) can be liberally applied and sterile disposable gloves placed over the fingers and hand, with the gloves securely sealed at the wrist. This type of dressing should be changed daily.

For burns of other parts of the body, Flamazine with gauze dressings, paraffin gauze dressing, or impregnated dressings with framycetin sulphate 1% (Sofra Tulle) with sterile gauze over can be applied. These dressings can be changed every three days, unless discomfort is experienced; if this is the case, change as often as necessary.

6   Abscesses, boils and infected cysts

Before an abscess, boil or infected cyst is ready for incision the patient should be encouraged to bathe the affected area at home, using hot saline water (one teaspoonful salt to one pint hot water), followed by an application of magnesium sulphate paste dressing. When the affected area is 'fluctuant' and 'pointing' an incision is made for the pus to be expressed. If the abscess or boil is very large and deep, the incision should be kept open to allow free drainage, which can be done by inserting ribbon gauze soaked in eusol and paraffin or saline and the dressing changed daily until drainage has ceased. In the case of a small abscess or boil after incision, a magnesium sulphate paste dressing can be applied and changed daily.

7   Ingrowing toenails

The correct way to cut toenails is straight across and not into the corners. Unfortunately many people do not do this and encourage the development of ingrowing toenails. By the time the patient comes to the surgery, the ingrowing toenail is usually infected, swollen, painful and discharging. In severe cases antibiotics may be needed, but the less severe can be treated daily with eusol soaks and a small wick of cotton wool soaked in eusol pushed between the nail and skin. The long term management lies in teaching the patient about nail cutting and the effects of tight shoes. Sometimes the nail is so distorted that wedge resection or nail removal will have to be done by the doctor under local anaesthetic. Persistent or recurrent problems may have to be treated by nail ablation which is a more formal orthopaedic operation.

8   Eye dressings

Some basic principles to be followed are:

1   Always tell your patient what you are doing.
2   Don't use an antiseptic spray on your hands.
3   Have everything ready.
4   Take care when using a torch, the patient may have photophobia.
5   Remember what a normal eye looks like.
6   Check the vision by enquiring from the patient.
7   Clean the lids thoroughly.
8   Don't touch the eye with the dropper or ointment tube, avoid drops going directly onto the cornea.
9   Don't put drops into the corner of the eye.
10   Always dry the eye when treatment is finished.

11   When covering the eye always fold the pad in half and place over closed lids.

12   If in doubt about the lids being kept closed don't use a pad at all.

Hotspoon bathing for eyes

1   Pad a wooden spoon to give thick pad.
2   Place a basin in a safe position at table height.
3   Fill a basin with boiling water.
4   Dip the padded spoon into the water and hold comfortably close to the closed lids allowing the heat to draw out the infection.
5   Continue until the water becomes cool. Take care not to touch lids with the padded spoon or burn the patient with steam.

EAR SYRINGING

Patients who need routine syringing of their ears for removal of wax should be encouraged to instil warm olive oil or cerumol into the ears three times a day for two days before syringing. Syringing should be approached carefully with hand-hot tap water. If the patient complains of pain or discomfort the nurse should stop syringing immediately and inspect the ear with the auriscope. No patient with a history of earache, discharge or perforation should have their ears syringed without an initial assessment by the doctor.

Equipment needed

Ear syringe or electric pulsed water action syringe
Receiver
Plastic cape and towel
Bowl with hand-hot tap water
Auriscope
Paper tissues

Method

(a)   Reassure the patient and explain exactly the routine of the procedure. Illustrate the type of sensation the patient will experience (e.g. when the warm water is pushed into the ear passage the feeling is one of diving into a swimming pool or swimming underwater—not a frightening feeling but slightly uncomfortable). Reassure the patient that the procedure should be painless but that if any pain is experienced the syringing will stop immediately.

Fig. 5.1   Leaflet on the use of eye ointments for patient instruction.

READ THIS NOTE BEFORE USING YOUR MEDICINE

NAME OF PREPARATION, DOSAGE INSTRUCTIONS   PATIENT'S NAME

PRESCRIBING DOCTOR   DATE

THE USE OF EYE OINTMENTS

1. Wash your hands before use.
2. When using a new tube for the first time, squeeze out a ¼" (about 1 cm) strip and throw it away.
3. To use:
   - (a) Tilt the head back slightly.
   - (b) With the lower lid turned down, gently apply a strip of ointment about ¼" (or 1 cm) long to the inner surface of the lid.
   - (c) Close the eye, and gently massage the lids for a few seconds.
   - (d) Remove any surplus ointment with a clean tissue.
   - (e) Vision may be blurred after applying this medication. Do not drive or operate machinery until vision is clear.

   If you find this difficult, it may be easier for someone else to do this for you.

4 Always replace the cap, and keep the tube in a cool place.
5. Avoid letting the nozzle of the tube touch the surface of the eye, or the lashes, or table tops, etc.
6. NEVER share your eye ointment with other people.
7. Discard any remainder when the treatment is finished, or after four weeks.

Further advice may be obtained from your Pharmacist or Doctor.

Pharmacist's Name:

Address:

Telephone Number:

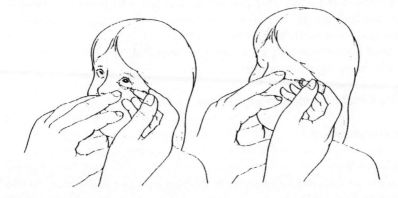

Illustrations by kind permission of Barrie & Jenkins 'The Action and Uses of Ophthalmic Drugs.'

Explain to the patient exactly what each piece of equipment is and how it works.

To some patients this procedure sounds and appears very frightening; it is important that the nurse shows great patience and reassurance towards each patient.

(b)   Patients should be seated with the plastic cape and towel around the shoulders for protection.
(c)   Examine the ears with an auriscope.
(d)   Ask the patient to hold the receiver firmly in place under ear.
(e)   Fill the syringe with water.
(f)   Draw the pinna backwards and upwards with the left hand.
(g)   Direct the water to the top and back of the auditory meatus using the syringe in the right hand (vice versa for left handed people).
(h)   Continue to syringe with care until wax is removed. Do not jam the nozzle tightly into the meatus.
(i)   Inspect the ears frequently with the auriscope during syringing.

MINOR SURGERY

With a well-equipped treatment room, minor surgery can be undertaken by the GP. This is more convenient to the patient, reducing the load on casualty and outpatient departments. The practice nurse is responsible for preparing the patient and instruments for minor surgery as well as giving the patient reassurance and comfort during the procedure. The role also involves the preparation of the site for minor surgery by cleaning the surrounding areas, shaving any hairs which may be troublesome and preparing the patient in the most comfortable and suitable position for the procedure. The instruments can be boiled in a water steriliser or autoclaved. The tray or trolley can then be laid up as a sterile procedure with sterile instruments, dressings, equipment and cleaning agents.

Minor surgery most commonly performed in the treatment room includes those items mentioned below.

1   Removal of cysts and papillomas

Necessary equipment

Top of trolley
Sterile equipment laid on sterile dressing sheet
Sterile disposable gloves

Scalpel blade holder and blade (size 15)
Spencer Wells forceps × 2
Toothed dissecting forceps
Plain dissecting forceps
Sponge holder
Scissors
Gallipot with cleaning agent
   (e.g. Cetavlon 1% Savlon or chlorhexidine)
Needle holder
Suturing material
   prepacked needle and thread, eyeless needled suture
   (e.g. Ethilon or Mersuture)
Sterile dressing pack containing dressing towels, cotton wool swabs,
   gauze swabs and gamgee pad

Bottom of trolley
Local anaesthetic (e.g. Xylocaine 1% or 2% prepared with sterile
   syringes and needles)
Elastoplast dressings as necessary
Specimen container with formol calcium solution for histological
   specimens

2   Opening infected cysts and abscesses

Necessary equipment

Top of trolley
Sterile equipment laid on dressing sheet
Sterile gloves
Scalpel blade and holder
Spencer Wells forceps
Sinus forceps
Gallipot with eusol and paraffin
Gallipot with chlorhexidine
Ribbon gauze
Dressing pack with cotton wool, gauze and padding

Bottom of trolley
Local anaesthetic (e.g. Ethylchloride spray)
Magnesium sulphate paste
Swab and culture medium
Elastoplast dressing strip as necessary

3   Removal or wedge resection of the toenail

Necessary equipment

Top of trolley
Sterile equipment laid on dressing sheet
Sterile gloves
Scissors
Scalpel blade and holder
Currettes
Spencer Wells forceps
Dissecting forceps
Dressing pack with cotton wool, gauze and padding
Gallipot with cleansing agent

Bottom of trolley
Rubber tourniquet
Local anaesthetic (e.g. Xylocaine 1% or 2% (NB without adrenaline)
   prepared with sterile syringe and needles)
Tubigauze (tubular gauze dressing) and applicator
Paraffin gauze dressing (e.g. Jelonet)

4   Suturing of injuries

Necessary equipment

Top of trolley
Sterile equipment laid on sterile dressing sheet
Sterile gloves
Needle holder
Suture material
   Prepacked single needle and thread (e.g. Ethilon, Mersuture)
Scissors
Toothed dissecting forceps
Spencer Wells forceps
Dressings

Bottom of trolley
Local anaesthetic (e.g. Xylocaine 1% or 2%)
Sterile syringe and needles
Elastoplast or bandage as necessary

5   Cuts not requiring suturing

Necessary equipment

Sterile gloves
Sterile steristrips
Dissecting forceps
Toothed dissecting forceps
Spencer Wells forceps
Scissors
Gallipot with Cetavlon 1% or chlorhexidine for cleaning
Dressings
Elastoplast or dressing strip

6   Removal of verrucae and warts

Necessary equipment

Sterile currettes
Dressings
Gallipot with cleansing agent
Local anaesthetic (e.g. Xylocaine 1% or 2%)
Sterile syringe and needle
Silver nitrate pencil
Electric cautery with attachments
Elastoplast dressing strip

7   Removal of a cervical polyp

Necessary equipment

Cusco vaginal speculum
Disposable gloves
KY Jelly
Long Spencer Wells forceps
Sponge holder
Cotton wool swabs
Silver nitrate pencil
Electric cautery with attachments
Anglepoise lamp
Specimen container with formol calcium 10% for histology and
    histology request form
Gallipot with cleansing agent

STERILISATION OF INSTRUMENTS AND DRESSINGS

Boiling

A water steriliser can be used for instruments and equipment (e.g. vaginal speculum, proctoscope, earpiece of auriscope, gallipots). Each item should first be soaked in a solution of Precept. These tablets can be ordered from the hospital pharmacy and contain sodium dichloriso-cyanourate. They dissolve rapidly in water to give a fast acting, wide spectrum disinfectant solution effective against vegetative bacteria, fungi, viruses and bacterial spores. They should then be scrubbed in running cold water to remove any dirt or blood before placing it into the steriliser. Boiling water will destroy most common non-sporing organisms in five minutes.

All surfaces to be sterilised in this way must be in contact with the boiling water throughout the boiling time.

Autoclaving

This process uses steam under pressure to sterilise instruments and equipment. The 'Little Sister' autoclave is most commonly used in the treatment room. This type of autoclave can be obtained in different sizes depending on size and types of instruments to be sterilised. The pressure in the autoclave chamber is raised to 30 pounds per square inch and a temperature of 135°C (370°F) is reached and held for three minutes. The length of time for this cycle is about eleven minutes. Each item to be sterilised should be first soaked in Precept solution and then scrubbed in cold running water to remove any dirt or blood before placing into the autoclave.

Dressings

High vacuum autoclave or hot air oven sterilisers are rarely used in general practice. The most economical and safe way of using sterile dressings is to use prepacked sterile dressing packs, ribbon gauze, gauze squares and cotton wool. These can be obtained on prescription for each patient through the local chemist and have usually been sterilised by irradiation.

TAKING OF SAMPLES

The taking of samples and specimens can be grouped into two categories:

1   Investigations undertaken at the pathology department
  (a)   Blood
  (b)   Urine
  (c)   Swabs
  (d)   Histology
  (e)   Faeces
  (f)   Sputum

2   Routine investigations undertaken at the surgery
  (a)   Urine
  (b)   Blood

INVESTIGATIONS UNDERTAKEN AT THE PATHOLOGY DEPARTMENT

1a   Blood

The practice nurse should be trained to take venous blood samples and some training programmes in hospital issue a certificate of competence for this. Practitioners will usually undertake the responsibility for training their nurse unless there is already a trained nurse, in which case it might be appropriate for her to show her colleague the techniques involved.

During the past few years the likelihood of contracting some serious illness, especially Hepatitis B or HIV infection (AIDS) has risen considerably. Therefore every care should be taken when extracting blood samples. A course of protection should be to wear rubber gloves when taking any blood sample (some authorities say two pairs). Many nurses will find this impractical and it certainly is very expensive for the practice. However, if there is the slightest doubt about exposing oneself to risk in taking a sample, full precautions should be taken. It is also important not to attempt to resheath the used needle in its container as the commonest cause of accidental injury when taking blood is from a needle stick. Both needle, syringe and container should all be thrown into a Sharps disposable bin after use. Pathology departments in different areas have their own specific requirements for samples, therefore it is the responsibility of the practice nurse to find out from her particular pathology department which samples of blood should be collected for each investigation. Table 5.1 lists the types of specimens and containers more commonly used in general practice.

As a general rule for most other blood tests not listed below 10 ml of clotted blood is taken. For any specialised tests arrangements should be made with the laboratory first.

Table 5.1 Specimens and containers commonly used in investigations in general practice.(These may differ from area to area.)

Type of investigation	Type of specimen and container	Request form
Haemoglobin	5 ml pink sequestrene bottle	Haematology
FBC and ESR	5 ml pink sequestrene bottle 1.5 ml mauve ESR bottle	Haematology
Biochemistry	10 ml clotted universal container	Chemical pathology
Blood sugar	2.5 ml yellow container	Chemical pathology
Paul Bunell or monospot screen for infectious mononucleosis	5 ml sequestrene of blood, film on a slide	Haematology
Antenatal blood for grouping and cross matching	10 ml clotted blood in universal container and two 4 ml sequestrene in pink containers	Antenatal
Rubella antibodies	10 ml clotted blood in universal container	Virology
Prothrombin time	2.5 ml of blood in a mauve prothrombin time container	General request
B12 and/or Folate	10 ml clotted blood in universal container	General request
Foetal haemoglobin	5 ml pink blood count bottle	Haematology
Malaria parasites	5 ml pink blood count bottle, thick and thin blood films	Haematology
Protein profile	10 ml clotted blood universal container	General request
RA latex fixation	10 ml clotted blood universal container	General request
Bone profile } included Liver tests } with chemical pathology	10 ml clotted blood universal container	Chemical pathology General request
Serum Lithium	10 ml clotted blood universal container Taken 12 hours (plus or minus 30 minutes) after an evening dose. Put times and amount of last dose	Chemical pathology General request
Serum Digoxin	10 ml clotted blood From 6–8 hours after oral dose—until just before next dose	Chemical pathology General request

Table 5.1   (Continued)

Type of investigation	Type of specimen and container	Request form
Serum Phenytoin	10 ml clotted blood Taken just before dose Put time and amount of last dose	Chemical pathology General request
Serum Carbamazepine	10 ml clotted blood Take before dose Put times and amount of last dose	Chemical pathology General request
Serum Phenobarbitone	10 ml clotted blood Take before oral dose	Chemical pathology General request
Serum Theophylline	10 ml clotted blood Take before oral dose	Chemical pathology General request
Serum Triglyceride	10 ml clotted blood Fasting	Chemical pathology General request
Serum Cholesterol + Lipids	10 ml clotted blood 12 hours fasting (if accurate result required)	Chemical pathology General request

High risk blood taking

If a patient is suspected of being in the high risk group of Hepatitis or HIV positive, blood must be taken with great care and sent to the pathology department in specially sealed container boxes with an 'At Risk' sticker in view.

1b   Urine: mid-stream specimen of urine (MSU)

An MSU is needed for culture and sensitivity. The patient is instructed on the method of collecting the urine specimen (the patient who collects the specimen at home is given an instruction leaflet with the sterile containers).

Urine samples—instructions to patient

1 Place a cleaned empty jar (e.g. 'jam' jar without lid) in a saucepan, cover with cold water, then bring to boil.
2 Pour off water and allow to cool.
3 Before urinating, *men* should wash the penis with soap and water, retracting the foreskin and drying carefully on a clean towel.

Women should wash the vulva with soap and water, using a cool but freshly boiled flannel, and drying carefully with a clean towel.

4 Start passing urine into the toilet bowl. When the stream is flowing freely, collect in the 'jam' jar.

5 From the 'jam' jar fill the screw top bottle containing *green* jelly culture. Pour the urine from this bottle into the *empty* screw top bottle. These bottles are obtained from the pathology department. Each culture bottle has an expiry date stamped on the side, so the nurse should check this before use.

6 Screw the caps of both bottles on firmly. Dispose of the 'jam' jar.

7 Allow the bottle containing the *green culture jelly* to stand *upside down* on its cap for 5 minutes.

8 Write your name clearly on the labels, and return both bottles to the surgery.

For patients who produce the MSU at the surgery a sterile dish is provided. Instructions are given for washing the vulva or penis with a soap solution (e.g. Cetavlon 1% or savlodil). The stream of urine is started into the toilet and the midstream is collected into the sterile dish provided. The nurse then pours the urine into the container with the culture medium and then transfers this to the clear bottle—the culture bottle is then turned upside down for five minutes. The containers are named and sent to the pathology department with the request form for the investigation required.

24-hour specimen of urine

All urine is collected for the complete 24 hour period in a large plastic container supplied by the pathology laboratory and returned to them after collection.

Pregnancy test

The urine tests are of the slide agglutination type which give an answer within a few minutes but are expensive to use in general practice, especially if the local laboratory gives a good service free. An early morning specimen of urine should be collected and sent in a sterile urine bottle with the pregnancy test request form. The first day of the last menstrual period is recorded on the form. The increasing sensitivity of this test means that it can be undertaken as soon as the menstrual period is overdue. However the result becomes more reliable when the sample is taken 7–10 days after the period is overdue.

1c   Swabs

Dry swabs

Dry swabs are taken from ear, nose, throat, infected wounds, eye, skin or rectum. The method of collection is by smearing the dry sterile swab across the infected area, collecting some discharge, then placing the swab across a frosted-ended slide labelled with the patient's name and returning the dry swab to the container. The specimen and slide should be despatched to the pathology department as soon as possible—if a delay is unavoidable the swab should be put into a transport medium (e.g. Stuarts medium).

High Vaginal Swab (HVS)

For HVS a swab is taken from the area of the cervical os. It is placed on to a named frosted-ended slide put into a culture medium and sent to the pathology department with a general request form.

Chlamydia testing for genito-urinary specimens (Elisa)

Elisa swabs and transport media and instructions are available from the pathology department. The swab used is made of cotton wool with plastic, wire or compressed paper stems, and the sample is collected from epithelial cells in the cervical os and not discharge.

Method of collection

  (a)   Female—endocervical swab.
        Remove any discharge. Insert swab into the endocervix and rotate using sufficient pressure to pick up epithelial cells. Withdraw without touching vaginal wall.
  (b)   Male—urethral swab.
        Remove any discharge. Insert swab 2–4 cm into the urethra and rotate using sufficient pressure to pick up epithelial cells.

Snap off cotton wool tip into Chlamydia Elisa transport medium and send to pathology department with a general request form.

Urethral swab

A swab taken from the urethra is plated onto a named frosted-ended slide and then put into transport culture medium.

Each swab is sent with the appropriate form giving history and request for investigation.

1d Histology

Cysts, lipomata and polyps which are removed by the doctor are immediately placed into a container of 10% formol calcium. Nail or skin scrapings are collected by cutting the affected nail or scraping particles of skin onto a cardboard slide container, the ends are sealed into an envelope and the patient's name attached. The appropriate history and request for examination should be sent with the specimen.

1e Faeces

Specimens of faeces are usually collected by the patient, at home, in a special container supplied with a spoon. The patient is instructed to place about six layers of paper into the toilet pan then pass the stool onto the paper and scoop a small section of the stool into the container with the spoon provided.

Tests for faecal occult blood can be obtained from the pathology department with full instructions for use.

1f Sputum

The patient is given a sterile sputum container to take home and advised to produce, after waking, an early morning sputum specimen. Ideally this specimen should be obtained *before* eating or drinking and *after* some deep productive coughing.

INVESTIGATIONS UNDERTAKEN AT THE SURGERY

2a Urine

Urine for the investigations shown in Table 5.2 is collected as a clean specimen.

2b Blood

(i) *Haemoglobin*

The level of haemoglobin can be estimated immediately by the use of a haemoglobinometer. The patient's finger is punctured with a sterilised steret, one drop of blood is dropped onto the raised canister

Table 5.2 Urine testing products and methods.

Name of product	Investigation for	Method
Uristix	Albumen, sugar	Dip reagent strip into urine and check colour against bottle label
Albustix	Albumen	As above
Clinistix	Sugar	As above
Clinitest	Level of sugar in urine (in diabetics)	To 10 drops water in test tube add 5 drops urine and 1 Clinitest tablet. Leave to foam for 1 min. When foam subsided compare colour with chart provided
Icotest	Bile	Place 5 drops urine on mat provided. Put one Icotest tablet on moist part and flow 2 drops water over. Result taken after 30 sec. Purple is positive result
Labstix	Sugar, albumen, blood pH, ketones, etc.	Dip reagent strip into urine. Compare colours with bottle label
Multistix	Specific gravity sugar, pH, bilirubin	Dip reagent strip into urine. Compare colours with bottle label.
Hema-Combistix	pH. protein glucose, blood	Dip reagent strip and check against label
Keto-Diastix	Glucose, ketones	Dip reagent strip and check against label
Hemastix	Blood	Dip reagent strip and check against label
Ketostix	Ketones	Dip reagent strip and check against label
Urobilistix	Urobilinogen	Dip reagent strip and check against label

of the glass slide, the blood is haemolised with the haemolising stick provided and the top slide applied. The prepared slides are then introduced into the haemoglobinometer to compare the level of colours and to estimate the haemoglobin.

(ii)   Testing for glucose level in the blood

Name of product	Method
Dextrostix	Apply large drop capillary or venous blood to stick to cover whole reagent area. Leave 1 min then wash blood off with water. Compare result with colour on bottle

There are also two blood glucose monitoring machines now available (Chapter 6).

(iii)   Erythrocyte sedimentation rate (ESR)

Send a blood sample to the laboratory (Table 5.1) or use Westergren tubes (Chapter 6).

REFERENCES

1   Newell R.L. and Turner J.G. (1985) *Orthopaedic disorders in general practice.* Butterworths.

Chapter 6

Equipment in the Treatment Room

The amount of equipment available in the treatment room will vary from practice to practice, but the nurse is responsible for upkeep of this equipment and knowledge about its correct usage. The usage and purchase of equipment will be considered in four groups:

1 Equipment for nursing procedures
2 Basic instruments
3 Specialised equipment
4 Miscellaneous equipment

Other suggested lists for equipment which can be used in the treatment room may be found in Jacka S.M. & Griffiths D.G. (1976) *Treatment Room Nursing* Oxford, Blackwell Scientific Publications.

1 EQUIPMENT FOR NURSING PROCEDURES

The equipment needed in a treatment room varies considerably according to the size of room available and volume of work performed by the practice nurse.

The necessary large equipment, such as couches, autoclave, desk, steriliser, chairs, lights, scales, height measure and trollies are checked and cleaned regularly by the practice nurse, who watches for any defects or items that may need replacing. These large items are either purchased by the doctor from the local wholesaler, wholesale chemist, or from mail order companies dealing with medical supplies. If the general practitioner is practising from a local authority health centre the large items may be rented from the authority concerned.

The smaller items of equipment needed for use in the treatment room are purchased by the general practitioner from the local chemist or wholesaler, items such as:

Ear syringe   Electric propulse ear syringe
Receivers   Eye visual chart
Eye glasses with pinhole   Ophthalmoscope

Orange sticks
Peak flow charts
Intravenous giving set for
    emergencies
Masks and gowns
Vaginal speculae and containers
Proctoscope disposable/metal
Auriscope
Stethoscope
Disposable gloves sterile/
    unsterile
Rubber gloves
Spatulae

Mini peak flow meters and low
    reading mini peak flow meter
Diets
Torches
Sphygmomanometer
Blankets
Pillows, pillow cases
Sheets
Towels
Armbands and tourniquets
Thermometers—oral and rectal
Nasal Speculum

2   BASIC INSTRUMENTS

The instruments required will be those necessary for minor operations, the removal of foreign bodies, dressing wounds, IUCD fittings. These can be purchased by the general practitioner from the local chemist, wholesaler or from a mail ordering company dealing with medical supplies and include:

Scissors, all sizes
Spencer Wells forceps, all
    sizes
Dissecting forceps
Tooth dissecting forceps
Splinter forceps
Scalpel blade holder and blades
Jobson horn probe
Mouth gag   ⎫ for emergency
Tongue forceps ⎭ tray
Suture removing blades
Aural and nasal forceps
Clip forceps

Suturing instruments (see
    Chapter 5)
Currettes
Silver probe
Instruments for IUCD fitting
    and checks (see
    Chapter 10)
Mosquito forceps
Suture removing scissors
Crocodile forceps
Splinter forceps

3   SPECIALISED EQUIPMENT

How much specialised equipment the practice nurse uses will depend on the interests of the doctors and, to some extent, on the accessibility to the facilities of a district hospital.

It is impossible to be totally comprehensive when compiling a list such as this but the more common specialised equipment which can be used by the practice nurse in the treatment room will be described.

Haemoglobinometer

A simple machine used for measuring the haemoglobin, it is of great value as a screening test in patients who might be anaemic. There are several models available. They all work on the colourimetric principle of contrasting the appearance of titrated blood when seen through a viewfinder with a known control and, once the colours are matched, reading off the haemoglobin level on a scale.

These machines are relatively inexpensive to buy and are quick and easy to use. They are only of limited value as they tend to be a little unreliable for accurate readings, but will certainly give an indication as to whether a patient should have blood sent to the haematological laboratory for further investigation. Each type of machine will have its own detailed instructions about operation with it.

Westergren ESR Tubes

The ESR (erythrocyte sedimentation rate) is a measurement of how fast the red cells collect as sediment in a capillary tube, and is a useful guide to serious pathology, or its absence, in a patient. It is a non-specific test in that a raised sedimentation rate could indicate anything from a respiratory infection to carcinomatosis but this would be a significant reading and the history and examination of the patient would usually indicate the next line of investigation. Special capillary tubes (Westergren) are required; citrated blood from the patient is drawn up into the tube and then the fall in level of the red cells over the course of one hour is timed. The result is then expressed as so many millimetres per hour. The normal range is 3–10 mm an hour for men and 5–15 mm an hour for women, but measurements just above this range are common and need to be interpreted carefully.

Microscope

The use of a microscope is mainly limited to looking for pus cells in urine when a urinary infection is suspected. The nurse will usually be familiar with a microscope from her past training, but she should refresh her knowledge on how to set up specimens and use the low and high power of the microscopes for effective use. This knowledge and instructions can be obtained by visiting the pathology department. The nurse will prepare the slide specimen for investigation so that it is ready for the doctor to see. Apart from its use in diagnosing urinary infections the microscope can be used to look for fungal hyphae in nail or skin scrapings, trichomonas vaginalis in a sample of vaginal discharge or for looking at blood smears.

The degree of use will be modified by the ready accessibility of a pathology laboratory but the opportunity to commence treatment before laboratory results are available should not be lost. There are, of course, many other uses for the microscope, but unless the doctors are particularly enthusiastic about its use or the practice is geographically isolated, the procedures mentioned above are the ones most likely to be performed.

Electrocardiogram (ECG)

At one time nearly all patients requiring an ECG had to be referred to hospital or the GP had to ask for a domiciliary visit from a consultant physician. Now many doctors and nurses entering practice are trained in the techniques of taking and interpreting the tracings of an ECG and expect to have this facility available.

The practice nurse re-learning to use the equipment can spend a day in the ECG department of the local hospital or be individually taught by the doctor. Essentially the ECG measures electrical potential in the heart muscle as it beats. The various electrical pathways are altered in muscle which has been damaged or where the heart is beating irregularly. It is these changes in electrical potential which give the tracing its characteristic appearance and enables the doctor to make a diagnosis about cardiac problems.

The nurse must be able to take a tracing if the practice owns an ECG machine and the following procedure is used.

1   The patient should be reassured and the procedure explained, particularly emphasising that it is painless and he or she will be unaware of any difference in the way they feel.
2   He or she should be lying on the couch, preferably a wooden framed one, as this reduces the chances of electrical interference with the tracing.
3   The chest, both wrists and ankles are exposed and the inside of wrists and ankles are smeared with a small amount of special lubricant which improves the electrical contract between the skin and the electrodes.
4   The wires from the machine are identified by colour coding (see below) and are fastened to the electrodes at wrists and ankles. The electrodes are clipped on to an elastic strap to secure them to the limbs.

Red   — Right arm   Green — Left leg
Yellow — Right leg   Black — Chest
White — Left arm

5 With the patient relaxed the tracing is begun.
6 First, it must be calibrated by pressing the appropriate knob on the machine. This enables the reader of the tracing to know the significance of the various wave heights.
7 Next leads I, II, III, aVR, aVL and aVF are measured in turn by moving the dial on the machine to the appropriate place. For each tracing of a lead let the tape run for about five or six heart beats unless the rate is very fast when more may be necessary. Certainly the length of each tracing need be no longer than 10–15 cm. Do not use vast quantities of tracing paper as it is expensive and yields no further information.
8 After this, the chest lead is attached using the suction cup and some more lubricant. It should be attached for the various chest (V) leads as shown in Fig. 6.1. Then leads V1 to V6 are each taken in turn.
9 When all the tracings have been taken the electrodes are unfastened from the wrists and ankles and the lubricant wiped off and cleaned. The patient can then get dressed.
10 Record the patient's name and the date at the beginning of the tracing.

Problems with the ECG machine

1 Not recording:
   (a) Check that the plugs are all pushed in properly and that the electricity is switched on.
   (b) Check that the machine has not run out of recording paper.
2 Interference with the ECG tracing. This is a common problem and can be caused by an assortment of extraneous sources such as other electrical equipment or the metal frame of the couch where the patient is lying. Loose elecrodes on the wrists and ankles or poor connections between the various electrical contacts and for the chest leads are also common causes of interference.

   If a patient is very anxious or restless this will cause other electrical impulses to be recorded which will interfere with the tracing.

   The equipment needs to be regularly serviced and the practice will have to make arrangements for this through the manufacturer or local hospital.

Fig. 6.1   Citing the ECG.

Lead I   = right arm and left arm
Lead II = right arm and left leg
Lead III = left arm and left leg
AVR   = right arm
AVL   = left arm
AVF   = left leg

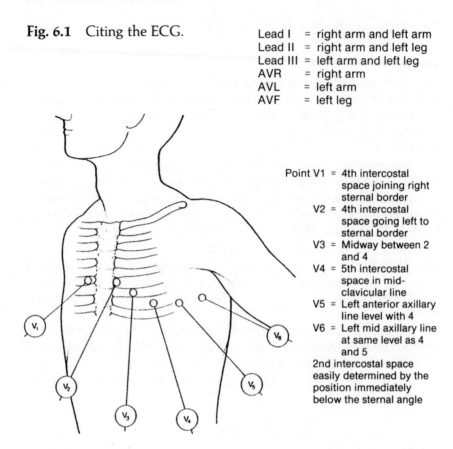

Point V1 = 4th intercostal
           space joining right
           sternal border
V2 = 4th intercostal
     space going left to
     sternal border
V3 = Midway between 2
     and 4
V4 = 5th intercostal
     space in mid-
     clavicular line
V5 = Left anterior axillary
     line level with 4
V6 = Left mid axillary line
     at same level as 4
     and 5
2nd intercostal space
easily determined by the
position immediately
below the sternal angle

The ECG tracing

An ECG tracing is not something that the nurse will have to be completely familiar with but an understanding of the activities makes the task more interesting. It is important that the nurse should be aware of the appearance of a normal ECG tracing so that if one she takes is grossly different she checks with the doctor before allowing the patient to leave the surgery premises.

Briefly, the wave formation of the tracing is caused as electrical depolarisation spreads across the heart muscle from the various nodes at which the electrical impulses originate. This gives the typical wave tracing shown in Fig. 6.2. However, this is modified by the position of the various leads which measure the depolarisation from different directions, and it is the reason why the various tracings of an ECG look different from different leads.

A few examples of common conditions are shown in Fig. 6.2.

If nurses are interested in further details about electrocardiography then there are many books on the subject.[1]

Cauterising equipment

The availability of cauterising equipment is helpful to any doctor undertaking minor operations in the treatment room. It is relatively inexpensive and the various cauterising heads can be used for removing warts or papillomata. If a wound is bleeding excessively the cautery can be used to seal identified bleeding points. Care must be taken not to burn the patient by careless application of the cautery to surrounding skin, especially if it has been anaesthetised so that the patient is unaware that it is happening.

The nurse is responsible for checking the equipment to see that it is working correctly and for cleaning the cautery heads. Care needs to be taken when doing this as they are quite fragile.

Peak flow meter

The peak flow meter was previously available as Wright's peak flow meter, which was a metal drum approximately 14 cm in diameter with a mouthpiece and a dial. The modern equivalent is a small plastic tube with a scale along the top and a moveable indicator; it is less expensive than the earlier model, light and portable and just as effective. The

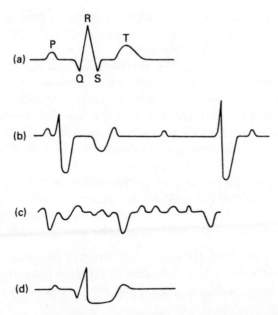

Fig. 6.2 Examples of ECG tracings. (a) Basic recording. (b) Complete heart block (conduction defect). (c) Atrial fibrillation. (d) ST depression in myocardial infarction.

mini peak flow meter can be supplied in a normal range for adults or a low range for children.

The principle of both is the same. They are used to measure the amount of air which a patient is capable of expelling forcibly from the lungs. It is not the volume of air which is measured, but the rate of expulsion. This is directly related to the elasticity of the lungs and the volume of air within the lungs and is measured in so many litres a minute. The normal range for an adult male of about 1.80 m in height would be 550–700 litres a minute. The normal varies depending upon height, weight, sex and age, but if in doubt there are tables provided with each instrument to give guidelines on this.

In the modern treatment of obstructive airways disease, and in particular asthma, the use of the peak flow meter is vital. Indeed, some doctors encourage asthmatic patients to keep one at home to use regularly, as a fall in the peak flow rate may be the first indication of the onset of a severe attack. Increase in medication at this time may abort or moderate the acute asthmatic attack. In the surgery it is used to monitor the progress of patients with obstructive airways disease and in particular the effectiveness of the various treatments available. To take the measurement the nurse explains to the patient as follows:

1   He or she should stand up to allow the maximum expansion of the chest.
2   The mouthpiece of the peak flow meter is held near the mouth with the plastic tube of the meter (modern design) held horizontally with the scale uppermost.
3   The patient expels all the air possible from his or her lungs and then takes a slow deep breath which expands the chest.
4   When the patient has taken as deep a breath as possible the mouthpiece is inserted between the lips and the patient forcibly expels the air from the lungs. It is important not to blow the air out but to forcibly contract the diaphragm in a 'huff' rather than a 'puff'.
5   If the procedure has been performed correctly the indicator will move out along the scale and the reading can be taken. The whole manoeuvre should be repeated several times, especially if the patient is unfamiliar with it, and the average reading taken.

In some patients with obstructive airways disease the readings will fall progressively as bronchoconstriction takes place and will increase again if a bronchodilator is used and then the reading repeated.

Nebuliser for inhaled medication

In recent years the use of the nebuliser for administering drugs used in various chest complaints has grown. The indications for use are discussed in Chapter 9.

The apparatus required to give nebuliser therapy consists of face mask/mouth piece, electric or foot nebuliser unit and the drug solution to be given, e.g. salbutamol sulphate BP (Ventolin Nebules 2.5 mg/ ampoule).

The nebuliser unit can be electrical or manual using a foot pump mechanism. Each machine comes with full instructions and it is simple and effective to use.

Glucose monitoring systems

There are two blood glucose monitoring systems now available for use in the treatment room. These machines can be purchased or may be given to the practice by a drug company:

1 The Reflolux II photometer offers easy and convenient determination of blood glucose and is used in conjunction with BM-Test-Glycemie strips.
2 The Glucometer also offers an easy and convenient test of blood glucose and is used in conjunction glucostix reagent strips.

Both these meters come with full instructions for use and are invaluable.

Electric pulse ear syringe

Within the last few years a new concept has been introduced to ear syringing techniques. The Propulse (Kitty) ear syringe has a gentle pulsed water action which speedily removes wax from ears. It is portable and can be operated off all electrical supplies, has a dialled pressure control combined with push button cut off valve, is sound proofed, insulated and is supplied with four colour coded interchangeable jet tips. The propulse system can also be used as an all-purpose lavaging tool, especially useful in wound debridement.

Each model can be supplied with either a foot or hand control switch.

Since the 1970s there has been a steady increase in the amount of equipment available to GPs, especially in the field of electrical and electronic measurements. How much of this equipment, from electronic sphygmomanometers to blood sugar measurement machines, is purchased depends on the availability of money and enthusiasm by the doctors of the practice.

Nevertheless, those doctors who prefer to use modern methods for the benefit of their patients will inevitably begin to acquire an

increasing amount of sophisticated equipment. It will be the responsibility of the practice nurse to familiarise herself with any new item,
know what it is to be used for and the principles of routine
maintenance for it.

STOCK-TAKING AND ORDERING OF SUPPLIES

It is the nurse's responsibility to equip and maintain the stock and
equipment in the treatment room. This should be checked weekly to
ensure that items do not run out at inconvenient times. Some items
can be prescribed, some have to be bought from the chemist or
wholesaler and others are provided free by the local authority or
hospital service. The following is a list of the various items which
might be used and an indication as to how to obtain them.

Items to be purchased from the local chemist

Dressings

Elastoplast dressing strips have to be purchased and so do specialised
items such as Mediswabs, tubigauze and applicators.

Cleansing agents

Including Savlon (ICI) hospital concentrate solution and Hibitane
solution for use in the treatment room.

Fixative for smears

Industrial methylated spirit can be obtained with a written request to
the chemist and is purchased by the practice.

Disposable items

These include wooden tongue depressors, disposable gloves, mouth-
pieces for the peak flow meter, disposable towels and sheets for the
couches.

Drugs

All emergency stock has to be purchased in the first place but can be
replaced by prescription when used or claimed for in the items liable
for reimbursement (e.g. influenza vaccine).

Dipsticks for urine testing

Various types are available for purchase, e.g. Uristix, Labstix, Ictostix Multistix or Haemastix.

Items available on prescription

Dressings and disposable items

Elastoplast and sterile dressing packs. Limited series of steristrips. Bandages and specialised dressings such as: tubigrip, paste bandages, tulle dressings, fixing tapes (micropore, blenderm, hypal), netelast, melolin, non-adhesive dressings, cotton wool and gangee tissue.

Lotions

Eusol, Cetavlon, chlorhexidine, Savlodil and saline, when being used for dressing.

Some dipsticks

Clinistix, Albustix, Diastix and Clinitest tablets are all prescribable for individual patients.

Special individual treatment

Special treatments such as antibiotic creams, powders, antibiotic impregnated gauze dressings, and other creams, sprays and ointments will have to be prescribed by the doctor.

Items available from the local authority or hospital pharmacy

The following items are available and can be ordered and obtained when needed. These items are free of charge for the doctor and nurse to use in the surgery.

Vaccines

Cholera and typhoid. In some cases Gamma Globulin, and Hepatitis B are prescribable.

In some areas all childhood vaccines can be obtained from the hospital pharmacy or health authority in single dose packages. These include:

Diphtheria, pertussis and tetanus (DPT)
Diphtheria and tetanus (DT)
Polio
Tetanus
Rubella
Measles
Immunoglobulin
Combined measles, mumps and rubella (MMR)

Gamma globulin injection

By specific request to the Public Health Laboratory for patients at risk travelling abroad, or can be prescribed.

Pathology specimen containers

From the pathology department or stores. Order on Pathology Stores request form.
   These include:

Blood bottles of all types
Urine bottles and culture medium
Swabs and cultures
Faeces containers
Hema-chek slide pak for occult blood
Slides, frosted ended and plain
Cytology spatulae and slide containers
Sputum containers for histology
Brown envelopes
Transport polythene bags
All request forms
Presept tabs for disinfecting
All needles and needle holders used in the Exe-tainer Evacuated method.

Diet sheets

May be available from the hospital dietician. There are also many good diet sheets which can be obtained from drug companies. (Appendix VIII.)

Disposable syringes and needles

Ordered from the Family Practitioner Committee.

Emergency trays

The practice nurse is responsible for the emergency trays in the treatment room. Each emergency tray should be laid up separately and clearly labelled. They should be placed in an accessible and known position so that all medical staff are aware of the contents and positions of the trays. The practice nurse maintains the level of emergency items, such as the following, on each tray. The items used on the emergency trays are purchased initially by the doctor and then those drugs used can be replaced by a prescription for the particular patient.

Eye tray

Most of the eyedrops listed can be obtained in separate sterile minims, which can be purchased from the local chemist or wholesaler.

Fluorescein 1%
Sodium chloride 0.9%
Chloramphenicol
Amethocaine 1%
Tropicamide
Mydrilate 0.5%
Atropine sulphate 1%
Castor oil

Eye pad and tape to hold in position
Eye bath

Laryngeal tray

Xylocaine laryngeal spray
Laryngeal mirror
Head mirror and strap
Methylated spirit lamp
Matches
Nasal forceps
Long throat forceps
Wooden spatulae
Swabs

Collapse tray

Brook Airway—all purpose model number 400, with clear instruction leaflet
Mouth gag
Airway
Tongue forceps
Intravenous giving set with normal saline and/or plasma substitute
Hydrocortisone 100 mg (Sodium phosphate or succinate) for intravenous or intramuscular use.
Aminophylline 250 mg in 10 ml for intravenous use.
Aminophylline 500 mg in 2 ml for intramuscular use.
Dextrose 50% in 25 ml for intravenous use.
Adrenaline 1/1000 in 1 ml for intramuscular use.
Chlorpheniramine (Piriton) 10 mg in 1 ml for intramuscular use.
Prochlorperazine (Stemetil) 12.5 mg in 1 ml for intramuscular use.
Prochlorperazine (Stemitil) 25 mg in 2 ml for intramuscular use.
Atropine Sulphate 600 mg in 1 ml for intramuscular or intravenous use.
Terbutyline (Bricanyl) 0.5 mg in 1 ml for intramuscular or slow intravenous use.
Diazepam (Valium) 10 mg in 2 ml for intramuscular or intravenous use.
Frusemide (Lasix) 20 mg in 2 ml for intravenous or intramuscular use.
Salbutamol (Ventolin) 0.5 mg in 1 ml for intramuscular use.
Tab. Chlorpheniramine (Piriton) 4 mg.
Tabs. Diazepam 2 mg + 5 mg.

REFERENCE

Hampton J.R. (1973) *The ECG made easy*. Churchill Livingstone.

Chapter 7

Immunisation and Preventive Care

The concept that the general practitioner should actually go out to his patients and offer services to improve their health is one which has only recently been accepted. It is now considered by the Royal College of General Practitioners and by those concerned with postgraduate training for general practice that preventive care is an integral part of primary care in the 1980s.

The practice record system must be organised in such a way as to meet this challenge. Of course there may be sources extraneous to the practice assisting in the preventive aspects of care. Until recently the government had a central bureau at Southport for collating results and sending out reminders to women throughout Great Britain who were due for cervical smears, but this proved inefficient as central records of this nature are inevitably incomplete. Some Family Practitioner Committees (Chapter 2) have now had their record systems computerised and are taking over the responsibility for administering the cervical smear recall service. However, this will not apply all over Great Britain and there are other aspects to preventive care besides cervical smears.

Amongst the many aspects are the immunisation programmes for children and it is vital that these are administered efficiently. Local health authorities assist in helping with the administration of calling up children under five for their immunisation schedule, but do not continue over this age when it is important (e.g. girls should have rubella vaccine at about eleven or twelve years old and tetanus and oral polio boosters should be given to all patients at approximately five-year intervals). The school medical service takes some responsibility for these activities, especially in relation to rubella, but yet again the uptake rate is poor and many children do not have the necessary immunisations by the time they leave school.

The practice nurse has a major role in administering the routine immunisation schedules of children. Local health authorities produce recall appointment cards and lists of immunisations, due twice monthly. The practice nurse or secretary is responsible for arranging to send the appointment card to the parent. When the child presents for the appropriate immunisation the nurse first confirms that there are no contraindications to giving the vaccine. The vaccine is administered intramuscularly into the upper leg for babies or the upper arm for older children. The polio vaccine is given on to the back of the tongue. The dosage for each vaccine should be checked with the manufacturers' instructions.

Some children experience a mild febrile reaction within 24 hours of having the triple vaccine. In these cases the parent should be advised to give mild analgesia together with tepid sponging in infants. Local swelling or redness at the site of injection is common and patients should be warned about this and reassured that it will settle within a short time. The practice nurse must be aware of the anxieties many parents have, particularly about pertussis vaccine, and be ready to reassure and advise them accordingly.

A RECOMMENDED PROGRAMME OF IMMUNISATION AND VACCINATION

At three months: Diphtheria, tetanus, pertussis and oral polio
At five months: Diphtheria, tetanus, pertussis and oral polio
At nine months: Diphtheria, tetanus, pertussis and oral polio
At 12–18 months: Measles. This will be replaced by the MMR (Measles, Mumps, Rubella) vaccine and should be given as soon as possible after the first birthday.
Pre-school: Diphtheria, tetanus, polio plus MMR vaccine if not already given. It should still be given if measles vaccine done or a history of measles, mumps or rubella was given previously.
10 years old   Booster tetanus and polio
12 years old   Rubella (unless MMR already given)
(girls only):
15 years old: Booster tetanus and polio

This is only intended as a guide and some programmes vary slightly. However, the principles for all these immunisation programmes (see following list) are the same.

1 It can only be started when the child is between three and six months old; until then the immune system is not sufficiently developed to produce the required antibody response. Indeed, some authorities would claim that children should wait until six months before starting immunisations for this reason.

2 The time is not specifically critical and if a child has missed an injection by a few weeks this does not matter. However, if there is a large lapse of time between injections then the whole course will have to be repeated if an adequate immune response is to be provoked.

3 Immunity to the diseases being immunised against will not begin immediately, and an important principle of epidemiology is that to protect the community from a specific disease a high percentage of that community will have to be immunised against it. The immunisation performed on a child is for its own good and for that of the population overall.

4 Many mothers have anxieties about the pertussis (whooping cough) vaccine as a result of adverse publicity about cases of brain damage, supposedly following administration of the vaccine. The risk of a severe reaction following immunisation for pertussis is about 1/100 000 provided the contraindications to immunisation (see below) are observed. Although the controversy still is debated, most authorities would now agree that the benefits outweigh the risks and one must not forget that whooping cough itself is not without its own mortality and morbidity. This fact is often conveniently forgotten by those who pursue the antivaccination campaign.

General comments

An excellent resumé of all the indications, contraindications and problems with immunisation is given in the DHSS booklet published in 1988.

This book explains that many conditions previously used as contraindications are *not* and include asthma, jaundice, prematurity and a history of allergy. Hypersensitivity to egg contraindicates influenza vaccine and anaphylactic reaction to egg contraindicates measles and mumps vaccine. All practices should have copies of this book readily to hand and use it for their own guidance and in counselling patients about vaccination.

Contraindications to specific vaccines:

Poliomyelitis

1 Immunological deficiency or immune suppression (e.g. cytotoxic drugs or leukaemia)
2 First four months of pregnancy
3 Febrile illness – postpone

4   Gastrointestinal symptoms – postpone
5   Sensitivity to neomycin.

Tetanus

None. Remember that antitetanus serum which used to provoke severe anaphylactic reaction is no longer used.

Repeated reinforcing doses of tetanus vaccine given unnecessarily for those who have been fully immunised within the previous five years can lead to hypersensitivity reactions.

Diphtheria

None, except if suffering from an acute febrile illness. Low dose vaccine *must* be used for persons over 10 years old.

Pertussis (whooping cough)

1   Fits in the child or neonatal cerebral damage
2   Close family history of fits
3   CNS disease — needs careful assessment of the pros and cons
4   Severe reaction to a previous dose of this vaccine
5   Intercurrent illness, but this means febrile illness rather than minor upper respiratory illness.

Measles

1   Immunological deficiency or supression
2   Hypersensitivity to the antibodies in the vaccine
3   Febrile illness
4   Active tuberculosis
5   Care in children with a history of allergy or convulsions although not a specific contraindication
6   Pregnant women
7   Not within 3 months of immunoglobulin.

Rubella

1   Immunological deficiency or suppression
2   Pregnant women
3   Thrombocytopenia
4   Hypersensitivity to antibiotics in the vaccine (neomycin, polymyxin)
5   Not within 3 months of immunoglobulin.

Measles/mumps/rubella

1 Children with acute febrile illness, vaccination should be deferred
2 Untreated malignant disease or altered immunity, those receiving immunosuppressive or X-ray therapy or high dose steroids
3 Children who have received another live vaccine by injection within three weeks
4 Allergies to neomycin or kanamycin or a history of anaphylaxis due to any cause
5 If MMR is given to adult women, pregnancy should be avoided for one month as for rubella vaccine
6 MMR vaccine should not be given within three months of an injection of immunoglobulin.

Hepatitis B

1 Hypersensitivity to previous vaccine
2 Pregnancy
3 Serious infection — may delay giving vaccine
4 Breast feeding mothers.

The success of an immunisation programme

A successful immunisation programme in the practice depends upon the enthusiasm of the practice staff responsible for administering it. In the best interest of the patient, the doctor, practice nurse and health visitor should work closely and agree on the practice immunisation policy together. These three members of the staff are most likely to be involved in counselling mothers who have anxieties about vaccination in general or one particular vaccine. It is unsatisfactory if the patient gets conflicting advice or anxiety provoking information unnecessarily from any one of the three.

Pertussis immunisation

A great deal of anxiety has been created in the last decade about this vaccination. Confusion first arose in the early 1970s when reports began to appear in the medical press about the possibility of brain damage to the child after pertussis immunisation. Biased reporting by some of the media together with conflicting medical opinions succeeded in reducing the immunisation rates for pertussis to very low levels in the mid- and late 1970s. The situation was not helped at this time by an ambiguous document on guidelines from the DHSS.

   In the last two or three years the position has become clearer and it is now possible to state some definite guidelines to those advising parents and patients.

1   The vaccine does protect the child from whooping cough and whooping cough itself is a serious illness. The last few years have seen several pertussis epidemics as a result of the fall in level of the herd immunity. At best the children and their parents have an unpleasant six or eight weeks while the disease runs its course and at the worst severe long term morbidity (or even mortality) can occur from lung damage or other complications.
2   There is a slight risk of cerebral irritation or more severe damage in a very small proportion of cases (100 000:1) but it is less than the problems caused by a clinical attack of pertussis.
3   A child with a history of an allergy or eczema can be given the vaccine.
4   Although febrile illness is a contraindication to vaccination at the time, many staff, who are unsure about the contraindications or unwilling to accept responsibility for decision making, will use excuses such as a minor 'cold' as a reason for not giving the vaccination. As many children are frequently catarrhal throughout the winter this means that the decision about vaccination gets postponed until it is forgotten. If in any doubt as to whether the child should have the vaccination always refer the matter back to the GP for a final decision.
5   Mild febrile reactions to the immunisation are common and only need to be treated symptomatically by the parent. A nodule on the site of the injection is also common and of no significance. In fact if both these matters are just mentioned to the mother at the time of the immunisation then it will stop her from worrying about them if they occur.

Rubella immunisation

With an active immunisation programme for rubella there is no need for any mother to give birth to a baby deformed as a result of her having rubella in early pregnancy. However, to date, at least one baby a week is born with this handicap. It is vital, therefore, that everyone associated with the responsibility for young girls between 11 and 13 years of age ensures that they have had a rubella immunisation.

It is insufficient to rely upon a patient's history of having had rubella earlier in childhood because immunological studies show that a history is unreliable as a guide to who is or is not susceptible to rubella infection. Many viral illnesses may mimic the rash of rubella and affect accurate diagnosis.

All girls between the ages of 11 and 13 years of age should be offered this immunisation. The school medical service will offer it but only a proportion of all those at risk will be picked up by this method as some children will be away from school, not tell their parents or avoid the issue in some way. The only reliable method is for the GPs and practice nurse to accept responsibility for this programme and have a record system such that they can recall the girls at, say, 11 years old to give them the vaccine. The record system should also enable them to know who has defaulted and ensure that these patients are contacted.

The length of time that immunity lasts is not yet known. It is a wise precaution for the nurse to take blood at the first family planning visit or antenatal attendance, to check on the immune status of the patient, who can then be given the vaccine at an appropriate time if she is found to be susceptible to infection.

Measles/Mumps/Rubella (MMR)

Four to five year old children attending for pre-school diphtheria/tetanus/polio booster can be offered MMR irrespective of history of measles or of measles vaccination. This 'catch up' campaign will reduce the number of rubella susceptible children entering school. The vaccine can be given at the same time as diphtheria/tetanus/polio in a different site. The vaccine can be given to children of any age.

Children who have a clinical history of having measles, mumps or rubella should be given the vaccination unless there is serological evidence of immunity to all three diseases. A single injection of 0.5 ml is given by deep subcutaneous or intramuscular route. No booster dose is necessary.

Minor side effects may be experienced, symptoms such as fever, rash, and malaise sometimes occur 5–10 days after vaccination. One per cent of children develop mild unilateral parotitis 3–4 weeks after vaccination.

Children with a personal history of convulsions or whose parents or siblings have a history of idiopathic epilepsy *should* receive MMR vaccine. Parents of these children should receive suitable advice for the prevention of febrile convulsions. Low dose measles specific immunoglobulin should not be given because of the theoretical interference with the acquisition of immunity to mumps and rubella.

Tetanus immunisation

The initial immunisation programme should begin with the triple vaccine (diphtheria, pertussis and tetanus) when the child is about six months old and the second dose given some six to twelve weeks later. One further dose a year after this completes the initial course and then a booster dose every five years is all that is required. Again certain life events (like starting or leaving school) are useful guidelines for continuing the immunisation programme. A good record system will show not only the current immune state of the patients but when the next booster dose is due.

There are no contraindications except in relation to rare immunological problems and no serious reactions. Far too many patients get unnecessary doses of vaccine, particularly if they are frequent attenders at a casualty department, and it is much better to keep the immune status 'topped up' by five-yearly booster doses and inform the patient that they need no further tetanus injections between these booster doses.

Polio immunisation

The disease, poliomyelitis, has been virtually eliminated by the success of the immunisation programme. However, if queries or anxieties arise about some aspects of the immunisation programme (such as with pertussis) this can have a 'spill over' effect and reduce the uptake of other immunisations. Constant vigilance must be kept to ensure that polio immunisation continues if this disease is not to recur.

There are three types of polio virus which are all included in the routine oral vaccine. They all produce specific immunity and as infection with one virus can interfere with the immunity of the other two it is important to give three doses of vaccine at least one month apart. Immunity is lifelong and repeat doses are given at school entry and leaving. These are not true booster doses but more a way of picking up those children who may have had an incomplete immunisation programme.

Polio vaccine should be offered to all parents at the same time as the first baby injection programme.

Measles immunisation

The epidemics of measles in children at about the age of five are no longer seen since the introduction of routine immunisation. This is done by giving a single injection of live attenuated virus which is supposed to give a long-lasting immunity in 95% of cases. However, it is common to find a proportion of immunised children getting a mild infection if the illness is going around the community.

The vaccine should not be given before the age of twelve months because of neutralisation by maternal antibodies, and a mild reaction consisting of a fever and occasionally a transient rash about the eighth day are common. Febrile convulsions may very occasionally occur but severe reactions such as encephalitis occur less than they do with the natural infection. If there is a history, or strong family history, of convulsions then the immunisation should be postponed until the age of three or four and a prophylactic anticonvulsant given for 16 days at the time of the immunisation. While egg sensitivity is a stated theoretical contraindication, the way in which the vaccine is cultured makes the likelihood of reaction extremely rare.

Note: Measles vaccine should only be given to children with the following conditions *with* an injection given simultaneously of human normal immunoglobulin (1.3 mg/kg body weight).

(a) History of convulsions
(b) Parental history of epilepsy
(c) Chronic disease of heart or lungs
(d) Serious failure to thrive.

Tuberculosis immunisation

The BCG vaccine has been available for many years and is offered to children around 11–13 years of age, but can be given at any age. It is preceded by a tuberculin (Heaf) test and only patients showing a negative reaction are vaccinated. The vaccine is given by the local authority school health nurse in the upper arm intradermally and occasionally the papule produced may break down and ulcerate. This is of no consequence and a dry dressing should be used to cover the site until it heals. Prior to administering a BCG vaccine an intradermal test (Mantoux) is performed to see that the patient is not hypersensitive to tuberculoprotein.

Hepatitis B vaccine

Hepatitis B has increased in the country since drug abuse has become commonplace.

Indications for giving

1 Health care personnel
2 Patient contacts from haemodialysis, haematology or oncology departments
3 Patients with increased risk due to sexual activities (e.g. homosexuals)
4 Plasma fraction workers
5 Drug abusers
6 Travellers to areas where hepatitis B is endemic.

The immunisation course consists of three injections given intramuscularly.

The second dose is given one month after the first and the third dose six months after the second dose. One month after the course is completed blood is taken to check if the patient is immune. On occasions a fourth dose may be needed to boost the immune state.

This vaccine is generally well tolerated with minimal side effects.

Influenza and immunisation programme

Many doctors have now introduced a specific influenza immunisation programme into their practice and, of course, the nurse plays a key role in this activity by being responsible for giving each vaccine. The establishment of a programme such as this requires careful thought and planning. The vaccine is obtained either by the practice buying directly from the drug company in bulk or by the doctor issuing individual patients with a prescription which they get from the chemist and then return for their injection.

There are some financial advantages to the practice in buying bulk vaccine as the GP can reclaim an item of service claim on this. However, if a GP only undertakes an influenza immunisation programme for money then he is probably better off expending his energies in other directions! He should believe that this is a service which it is desirable to offer to his patients.

Patients who would be offered the vaccine by the doctor include those over 65, and special cases such as patients suffering from severe chest or heart disease and diabetese. In addition, it is important that the staff, especially the medical personnel, have the vaccine. Other patients may also request the vaccine if they know of the practice policy and it is difficult to refuse in these circumstances because it is a preventive care activity, but the recent DHSS guidelines specifically state that only 'at risk' patients should be offered the vaccine.

There are two influenza viruses, A and B, but whereas most viruses are antigenically stable these are constantly altering their structure. This is the reason why it took so long to develop an effective vaccine and why some patients will get influenza despite having had the vaccine.

The World Health Organization issues guidelines annually about what is the most likely effective vaccine to be used in a particular year.

Establishing the programme

The doctors and nurses should decide who are going to be immunised against influenza and then these patients can be identified from the age/sex and disease registers (see Chapter 3). The practice can either send for the patients concerned offering them an influenza immunisation or wait for them to turn up in surgery. If the latter course is taken not all those at risk will be covered and the whole process will take much longer. The best time to start the programme is in late September or early October. The bulk of the immunisations should be given before the end of the year to protect patients in the early part of the following year when influenza epidemics are most likely.

The vaccine should be given by the nurse by subcutaneous or intramuscular injection into the upper arm. The patient must be reassured of the minimal side effects which may be experienced (e.g. localised pain and redness may occur at the site of injection, febrile symptoms may also be present for 24 hours). These symptoms can be treated systematically by the patient with analgesia. The immunisation will need to be repeated annually, possibly with a different strain of virus depending on the current likely infections.

The vaccine may be expected to protect the patient from influenza 10–21 days after administration.

The practice nurse should only give this vaccine while a doctor is on the premises and adrenaline must be readily available.

OVERSEAS TRAVEL

Many patients are now travelling overseas for business and pleasure. They will make enquiries about the various immunisations required and it is important for the practice nurse to know the current requirements and to be able to work out an immunisation programme for an individual who may need several injections. The newspaper *Pulse* has a pull-out supplement which is regularly updated for requirements and this is probably the most accessible source for most nurses. This list of requirements is issued by the World Health Organization.

Cholera immunisation

Some countries still require an international certificate of vaccination against cholera. Although the vaccine produces some individual protection for up to six months it does not prevent spread of the disease which is closely related to the standards of hygiene in practice.

Age	First dose (given subcutaneously or intramuscularly)	Subsequent doses (given intradermally)
1–5 years	0.1 ml	0.1 ml
5–10 years	0.3 ml	0.1 ml
Over 10 years	0.5 ml	0.2 ml

Primary vaccination consists of two doses ideally one month apart. The interval can be reduced to seven days, although this makes the immune response less effective. The immunity is short lived, so booster injections should be given every six months to people who continue to be exposed to the risk of contacting this disease.

Typhoid immunisation

The use of typhoid vaccine is a guarantee of immunity to the disease only if careful hygienic precautions are followed. The nurse can give and advise on these precautions by suggesting the patient avoids eating salads, unwashed or unpeeled fruit, uncooked food or drinking non-sterile water.

Most severe reactions can be avoided by giving 0.1 ml of the vaccine intradermally but it is not certain if this produces as satisfactory an immune response as 0.5 ml subcutaneously as usually recommended. For primary immunisation against typhoid two doses are normally required, the first dose of 0.5 ml is given deep subcutaneously followed by the second injection of 0.1 ml given intradermally four to six weeks later. If exposure to risk continues a further reinforcing dose of 0.1 ml intradermally is given every two to three years. When reaction does occur it consists of swelling and pain at the site of the injection and sometimes a systemic reaction with fever and general malaise for up to 48 hours. These symptoms can be treated by the patient with analgesia and rest.

Age	First dose (given subcutaneously or intramuscularly)	Subsequent doses (given intradermally)
1–10 years	0.25 ml	0.1 ml
Over 10 years	0.5 ml	0.1 ml

Primary vaccination consists of two doses ideally 4–6 weeks apart although if the time is restricted between the two injections an interval of not less than 10 days will be sufficient. However, the value of the second injection is uncertain.

Yellow fever immunisation

The individual should be informed by his travel agent if this vaccine is required (Africa and South America). If the patient is not using a travel agent the practice nurse has a current list of vaccinations and immunisations needed for travelling abroad. The practice nurse will not give it as it can only be given at designated centres. Her responsibility lies in knowing where her local designated centre is. These centres are run by the local health authority, most have clinics once or twice weekly so an appointment should be made for the patient with the clinic. The vaccine should not be given to anyone sensitive to egg, polymyxin or neomycin, under nine months of age or pregnant, but otherwise there are no contraindications and reactions are rare. A fee is usually charged by the centre.

Smallpox immunisation

Smallpox vaccination is not done routinely as the disease has been eradicated and a certification of smallpox eradication declared the world free of smallpox in 1979 and this was ratified by the WHO in 1980.

There is thus no indication for smallpox vaccination for any individual except, possibly, in some cases of laboratory workers using pox virus.

Malaria prophylaxis

Patients frequently seek advice about prophylaxis against malaria. While there is no immunisation against it this would seem an appropriate place to include guidelines on this. To really understand the prophylaxis thoroughly one must be aware of the different forms of malaria, the life cycle of the parasite and the current status of drugs in use, as resistance to treatment is becoming a problem. These aspects are beyond the scope of this book but may be obtained from any textbook of medicine.

From the point of view of prophylaxis two drugs are in common use and they should be taken from the day before travelling until at least four weeks after leaving the area. The choice of drug lies in either taking a once daily dose of proguanil (Paludrine) or a weekly dose of chloroquine. Other drugs are replacing the older drugs in areas such as South America where drug resistance is occurring.

Advice may be obtained from the London School of Tropical Medicine and Hygiene on the drugs currently recommended for the different areas of the world. The World Health Organization also issues a monthly format to follow for the different areas and drugs recommended for malaria prophylaxis. These drugs can be purchased over the counter at the chemist by the patient after receiving a private prescription from his doctor. A suggested format for a prescription of this nature is shown in Appendix I.

Human normal immunoglobin

This can be used in the protection of susceptible contacts of infectious hepatitis patients or for those travelling to countries where exposure to infection is likely. The vaccine can be ordered from the Public Health Department or obtained on prescription. Ideally blood should be taken first to check if the patient is immune to hepatitis A and B to see if the vaccine is needed.

The dosage for patients travelling abroad:

Age	Abroad under 2 months	Abroad over 2 months
Under 10 years	0.125 g	0.25 g
Adult dose	0.25 g	0.50 g

General comments

It is a good principle to encourage patients to start their particular immunisation programme well in advance of their travel if at all possible. Try not to give more than one immunisation at a time, or at least separate individual vaccinations by a few days. The more time that can be left between the first and second dose (up to four weeks) the better. Use the opportunity to give the patient general advice concerning hygiene and eating habits while abroad and perhaps advice on some basic simple medication which they can take with them (e.g. lomotil). Remember that prescriptions cannot be issued for illnesses that have not taken place just 'in case'; this does not stop the patient from ensuring that they have an adequate supply of any regular medication which they take. It is important to try and avoid running out of medical supplies when abroad as the drugs available may not necessarily be comparable with the British variety. These comments also apply to the oral contraceptive pill which patients may not look upon as a regular medication.

Any patient requesting an international vaccination certificate for smallpox or cholera can be charged for this as the issue of certificates (as opposed to giving the vaccine) is not covered by the GP's terms of service. Also a charge can be made for a private prescription for malaria prophylaxis. These are signed by the doctor and stamped with the GP's name and address. A private certificate may be issued if patients request verification of other vaccinations given to them.

OTHER ASPECTS OF PREVENTIVE CARE

Earlier in this chapter the principles of preventive care were mentioned and the fact that GPs and nurses should regard themselves as responsible for the care of their practice population in preventive, as well as curative, terms. This has wide ranging implications and a great deal of the routine workload of this decision will fall upon the practice nurse. The need for special clinics such as obesity or antenatal are discussed in Chapter 11. Other aspects include developmental assessment in young children or cervical smears in women.

Developmental assessment

There has become increasing awareness of the need to screen young children for certain specific abnormalities, especially vision and hearing. In addition their general developmental progress is also assessed.

The GP may do his own developmental assessment, or one of the partners may have a special interest in children and do it all. In some areas this responsibility may be undertaken by the local health authority. The health visitor has major responsibilities for children under five, but occasionally the practice nurse may be involved in organising a regular developmental assessment session in the practice and she may, indeed, combine it with an immunisation programme at the same time. A guide to the suggested programme for certain assessments in children under five is shown below.

In *Healthier Children—Thinking Prevention* (Royal College of General Practitioners 1982) the whole aspect of preventive child care is discussed and the case made for some form of routine screening in childhood. The paper encourages 20 important points to be checked during the growth from babyhood to adulthood and it might be worth a practice incorporating such a checklist for patients in its record system. The recommendations are divided into three categories.

Prebirth

1   Contraception
2   Breast feeding
3   Discouraging smoking
4   Antenatal care

At birth

5   Chemical screening, e.g. phenylketonuria
6   Congenital dislocation of the hips

7   Maldescent of the testes (boys)

After birth

8   Polio immunisation
9   Tetanus immunisation
10   Diphtheria immunisation
11   Pertussis immunisation
12   Measles immunisation
13   Hearing
14   Squints
15   Visual acuity
16   Colour vision
17   Rubella immunisation (girls)
18   Scoliosis
19   Discouraging smoking (child)
20   Contraception (child)

Cervical smears

The routine screening for carcinoma of the cervix by taking a cervical smear has now become recognised practice. However there are still many aspects of this activity about which matters are not clear (e.g. while some women show dysplasia in the cervical cells it is not known what proportion of these go on to develop carcinoma *in situ*). Dysplasia is the early sign of abnormal change in the cell and may only be managed by repeat smears at intervals suggested by the pathology laboratory. The degree of the severity of the change is rated on a scale (CIN 1-111) and the laboratory will indicate the stage at which referral should be made to a specialist or suggest the interval before repeat. Carcinoma *in situ* is premalignant change in those cells and can be dealt with by local removal of the tissue concerned (cone biopsy) or by laser treatment. Similarly while most women will be treated at the stage of carcinoma *in situ* it is known that this condition may persist without frank malignant change.

The high risk factors increasing the chance of developing carcinoma of the cervix, are:

1   Poor personal hygiene
2   Multiple partners
3   Commencing intercourse at an early age
4   High parity
5   Low social class
6   Smoking

Several of these factors are found in patients who will not routinely present themselves for a cervical smear. The middle class low parity woman is not the one at risk from these factors, taking the opportunity to have a smear if requested or if she believes that it is time that it was repeated. Persuading the patients at risk to have a smear regularly is a real challenge to the practice and may require the combined efforts of the practice team to achieve success.

The practice record system must be designed to indicate when a woman last had a smear and have a recall system to remind the staff of when the next smear for a patient is due (see Chapter 3). At present a general practitioner can claim payment for cervical smears performed on women over 35 or who have had three pregnancies (including termination or abortion). These payments can only be claimed at five-yearly intervals on form FP74.

There is controversy over how frequently women below this age or who are on oral contraceptives should have a cervical smear. Certainly it is possible for a woman to have carcinoma of the cervix in her twenties, and it is probably sufficient to commence taking routine smears within a year or so of a woman starting sexual activity at an interval of about every three years. This aspect is discussed further in the chapter on contraception.

OTHER SCREENING ACTIVITIES

There will be a limit to the number of screening activities which can be undertaken by a practice and continue also to see patients who are ill! The partners must decide their priorities in this matter but there are certain principles which are important in considering routine screening.

1 The condition must be treatable.
2 It must have a recognised latent period during which it can be detected, e.g. diabetes or hypertension.
3 The test must be simple, cheap and reliable.
4 The return must be cost effective in terms of money and manpower.

Screening can be undertaken on a major formal basis (e.g. calling up men between 40 and 60 years of age to have their blood pressure measured). On the other hand it can be opportunistic, such as taking blood pressure and testing the urine of patients when they are present for other reasons. The latter is less expensive in terms of money and time but it will take longer to cover the practice population and require a certain amount of dedication on the part of doctors and nurses not to miss an opportunity. Either way it requires:

1   An attitude of mind on the part of the practice staff towards the principles of preventive care
2   Records to indicate when an action was last taken or if it has been taken at all
3   Recall systems which can only operate with an age/sex register
4   Full agreement from all concerned that the activity is worthwhile, cost effective and efficient. This means that the systems must be reviewed from time to time
5   The completion of all appropriate claim forms so that where money can be earned it is. On many occasions activities will be undertaken without attracting payment (cervical smears on women under 35) but good business principles dictate that opportunities should not be missed when they arise.

These are the attractions and challenges of preventive care and no general practice in the 1980s can consider it is up-to-date if these matters are not given serious regular consideration to continue to improve the service to patients.

REFERENCES

DHSS (1980) *Immunisation against Infectious Disease*. HMSO.
RCGP (1982). *Healthier Children Thinking Prevention*.
Dawood R. (1986) *Travellers Health*. OUP.

Chapter 8

Emergency Procedures

From time to time life-threatening crises will occur in the treatment room and the nurse must be confident and competent to deal with these when they arise. In addition she will sometimes find herself as the only medically qualified member of staff on the premises when an emergency call is received. She will be expected to assess the degree of urgency of the request, and assist the reception staff in deciding what course of action is to be taken if a doctor is not immediately available for advice.

GENERAL PRINCIPLES

In the event of emergencies in the treatment room, the practice nurse must always be mindful of the basic principles of first aid. M. Skeet[1] states that,

'First aid is given to:
  sustain life
  prevent the condition from becoming worse
  promote recovery
The person rendering first aid must:
  assess the situation
  arrive at a diagnosis for each ...
  give immediate and adequate treatment, bearing in mind that a casualty may have more than one injury and that some ... will require more urgent attention than others
  arrange without delay for transport ... to a hospital according to the seriousness of the condition'.

While the practice nurse is unlikely to encounter situations involving multiple casualties and may even find the individual crisis a rarity, nevertheless she must always be aware that these can occur and keep her own basic first aid skills up-to-date. The following general principles always apply:

1 Maintain a professional attitude of calm, despite how you might feel inside

2   Whatever the situation, whether on the premises or a telephone call, try and collect relevant information and defuse the anxiety of relatives and friends of the patient. Take charge confidently, resisting any hasty course of action because of the pressure of anxiety of those around you

3   Life-threatening emergencies obviously call for immediate action—for example:
     (a)   asphyxia
     (b)   sudden loss of consciousness
     (c)   profuse haemorrhage

4   Other situations—and by far the greater majority—will be for practical purposes unaffected whether the action be taken immediately or within, say, half-an-hour. For example, if someone on the telephone is with a patient who has collapsed, possibly with a stroke, then provided instructions are issued about putting the patient in the recovery position then no other immediate help is going to make a difference to the outcome. Indeed one often finds that patients are recovering from a variety of 'collapses' by the time medical help arrives at the scene

5   In urban surroundings it will probably be easy to obtain the help of the ambulance service if the doctor is not immediately available, but in rural locations this will be more difficult. In either case the service is expensive and hard pressed so the nurse still needs to make a calm assessment as to whether to dispatch an ambulance or not. It will not enhance the reputation of a practice to use the ambulance service casually.

COMMON EMERGENCIES IN PRACTICE AND FIRST AID MANAGEMENT

Asphyxia

Blockage of the patient's airway so that the brain is rapidly starved of oxygen is probably the most urgent of all general practice emergencies.

Asphyxia can occur in many ways, from inhalation of a foreign body to crush injuries in a serious accident, but the basic principles for treatment remain the same, and a sucker should be available in the treatment room to clear the airway. In addition, a Brook Airway and ordinary airway as used in anaesthetics should be part of the treatment room equipment.

Diagnosis

The history may make this obvious (e.g. the mother sees a child swallow a marble and the child then goes blue and chokes). However, in other situations such as the unconscious patient it may not be so obvious immediately.

An asphyxiated patient always loses consciousness quickly and face and extremities become cyanosed. If action is not taken then the heart soon ceases to beat and after this the chances of resuscitation are slight.

Treatment

Urgent action is essential. If asphyxia is due to an inhaled foreign body then several manoeuvres may help.

Children   Infants and babies should be held upside down by the feet and hit smartly between the shoulder blades. Children may be draped face down over the first aider's knee or arm and smacked firmly between the shoulder blades. This will frequently dislodge the offending object, the child will gasp, return to its normal colour, starting crying and all will be well.

Adults   Feel in the mouth to make sure that obvious obstructions, such as dentures, are not present and begin mouth-to-mouth resuscitation, or preferably use a Brook Airway (see Fig. 8.1). It is not proposed to go into the details of mouth-to-nose or -mouth resuscitation as many nurses learn this during their training and the procedures are well described in first aid books.

There is one procedure that is worth mentioning because it is not universally known. This is the Heimlich manoeuvre and is performed on an adult who has choked on food. The history is frequently that the patient suddenly collapses at the dining table and cases of asphyxia due to obstruction of the airway by a piece of meat have been mistakenly diagnosed as a fatal heart attack.

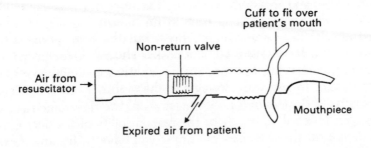

Fig. 8.1   A Brook Airway.

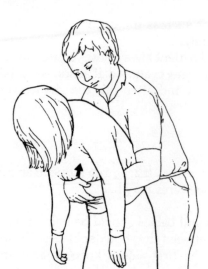

Fig. 8.2   Heimlich manoeuvre.

Heimlich manoeuvre   Any patient who collapses whilst eating should be assumed to have choked until proved otherwise. The first aider stands behind the patient and supports the back against his or her own chest and abdomen. The first aider, with arms clasped around the chest of the patient below the ribs, clenches the fists below the xyphisternum. A sudden inward and upward movement should be made with the arms to jerk the clenched fist up under the sternum (see Fig. 8.2.). This is an effective way to drive air forcibly up the airway and will often dislodge the offending obstruction, after which the patient will quickly recover.

The unconscious patient

All unconscious patients should either be laid on their back with the head extended and an assistant holding the angle of the jaw extended to prevent the tongue falling back in the mouth (see Fig. 8.3.), or turned into the 'recovery position', three-quarters prone with the face turned to one side (see Fig. 8.4.). This position is advised for any patient who might vomit while unconscious, to prevent inhaling the vomitus. It is preferable to insert an airway into the mouth if one is available.

The cause of the loss of consciousness should be determined as soon as possible. This will normally be the responsibility of the doctor, but if one is not on the premises the nurse will have to try and do this herself. Try and get any relevant history from relations or friends accompanying the patient or from the patient's notes (e.g. he or she

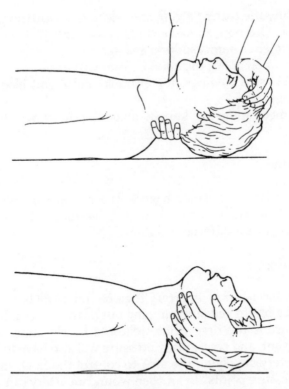

Fig. 8.3   Extension of the patient's neck to maintain an airway.

may be a known epileptic). Check the pulse, blood pressure and pupils as a baseline for determining changes in these over the course of the next few minutes. If there is any question of the cause being a deliberate overdose of medication and/or alcohol, make a note of any relevant treatment and check the patient's belongings to see if any medicines are being carried with them (e.g. if a bottle of glyceryl trinitrate was found in the pocket this would strongly support a presumptive diagnosis of a heart attack).

If the patient cannot be roused, and no medical aid is available, then it is best to call the emergency services for an ambulance. Write a note

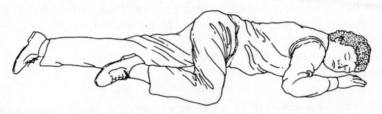

Fig. 8.4   Recovery or coma position.

to accompany the patient giving any relevant information which you have found. This note should include (if known):
(a)   The patient's name, address and age
(b)   Information about the episode from witnesses
(c)   Any physical findings, for example, pulse and blood pressure readings
(d)   Any medications or known medical history which might be helpful

Haemorrhage

Most cuts and minor haemorrhage will soon stop if simple pressure is applied with a pad to the site of the bleeding. However certain situations require a different solution.

Arterial bleeding

If an injury has severed an artery then bleeding will be profuse. The blood will be bright red and pumping out of the wound. In this case, local pressure is the first action, followed by elevation of the limb where relevant, and occasionally pressure will also have to be exerted over the artery supplying the area to control the flow, the so-called first aid 'pressure points'. In an open wound an artery can sometimes be seen to be bleeding—if so, then the direct application of a Spencer Wells artery forceps to the cut end is the most effective way to control the bleeding.

Varicose veins

Occasionally patients with varicose veins will knock their legs and puncture the veins. The bleeding is impressive but, of course, is venous so the blood is darker, slower flowing and not pumping out. The wound itself may be almost invisible but still may bleed copiously. The treatment is simple—lay the patient down, put a pad on the wound, elevate the leg and the bleeding will cease immediately. After the patient has been lying flat with the leg elevated for half-an-hour, the nurse puts a firm pad and bandage on the leg before allowing the patient to walk.

Haematemesis

Haematemesis is unlikely to occur in surgery but occasionally a call may be received. Most episodes of vomiting of blood are significant but not desperately urgent, unless a large and obvious quantity has been produced, when the patient will quickly become shocked with a weak, rapid pulse and a fall in blood pressure. This call requires urgent hospital admission, but more minor cases can be reassured and rested until a doctor can be contacted to assess them. If the practice nurse receives a telephone call or encounters a case requiring urgent hospital admission and there is no GP present, an ambulance is called, stating the nature of the emergency and giving the casualty department the information mentioned earlier.

Swallowed blood from the posterior nasal space is often mistaken for a haematemesis and this cause should be considered. Taking an accurate history usually clarifies this issue.

Melaena

Bleeding within the bowel can often be overlooked in a patient who collapses with no apparent cause. A more common presentation is an unexplained iron-deficiency anaemia in which case one might be asked to do an occult blood test on the faeces.

For an occult blood test, a specimen of faeces is collected (see method of collection of faeces, Chapter 5). To reduce the chance of a false positive result the diet must exclude all red meats and green vegetables for at least three days before the test is to be carried out. However, this is rarely practical but the occult test is still useful. The traditional black tarry stool of the severe melaena makes the diagnosis easy for the doctor or practice nurse. Patients with frank melaena need hospital admission for further investigations.

Epistaxis

Nose bleeds are very common, particularly in children, and the nurse must be competent to handle them. The first line of treatment is to reassure the patient and sit him or her down and loosen tight clothing around the neck. The nose is pinched firmly between finger and thumb for a *timed* ten minutes, while the patient breathes through the mouth, the head is tilted slightly forward and an ice pack can be applied to the bridge of the nose. A towel or bowl on the patient's lap helps to protect the clothing.

This action will stop a very high proportion of nose bleeds in children and some in adults. An clot which has formed at the nostrils should be left alone and not blown out as this will restart the bleeding. In fact the nose should not be blown hard for as long as possible, perhaps 12–24 hours. Recurrent nose bleeds in children are often due to a dilated single capillary in the lower part of the nasal septum and in these instances the GP may want to cauterize the vessel. This is done using phenol BPC on cotton wool on an orange stick after anaesthetising the area with local anaesthetic. It is very important to be careful when using phenol as it destroys the tissue and is extremely caustic. The practice nurse's role is to prepare, care for and reassure the patient and prepare the phenol, cotton wool and orange stick and local anaesthetic solution ready for the doctor to use. The patient must be told not to blow the nose for at least 12 hours and to avoid strenuous exercise and very hot baths for a similar length of time.

In adults the bleeding sometimes occurs from higher up the nose and may be precipitated by rupture of a small arteriosclerotic capillary. Hypertension must be considered as a cause of nosebleeds in adults so it is always worth taking the blood pressure and pulse. This becomes a useful item of information anyway if the haemorrhage is profuse and repeated as occasionally adults need hospital admission if the bleeding will not stop.

If the simple squeeze technique does not stop the bleeding then this may be repeated several times. When it is obvious that the bleeding is not going to stop then the nose will need to be packed by a doctor using long forceps and a sterile nasal packing. The nurse's role is to prepare the sterile ribbon gauze packing and sterile forceps for the doctor to use and to reassure and care for the patient. This packing should be carefully removed after 24 hours by the nurse with sterile forceps. An alternative simple packing is sterispon which is a synthetic sponge pack easily inserted and which reabsorbs without having to be specifically removed. The practice nurse can insert this packing without supervision from the doctor if she is trained to do so.

Other causes of collapse

Simple faint (Vasovagal attack)

Probably the commonest cause of a patient collapsing in the treatment room is a faint. If a patient should faint from an obvious cause such as venepuncture then remove the needle and get the patient flat as quickly as possible. If he or she was sitting in a chair then it is possible that the nurse will have to lay the patient on the floor as he or she will be too heavy to get on to a couch without assistance.

Most patients who feel faint get some warning of this, becoming pale, complaining of nausea and sweating, and making a comment to this effect. If the head of the patient is quickly lowered between their knees for a minute or so while sitting on the chair this will often prevent an actual faint from occurring. Talking with, and reassuring, the patient will also help to prevent a faint as anxiety and imagination play a major role in precipitating a vasovagal attack in this situation. A patient who has collapsed from a simple vasovagal attack will quickly recover when horizontal and this is a useful diagnostic pointer to the cause of the collapse if the nurse is unsure.

Epilepsy

A generalised seizure such as *grand mal* can be frightening for both patient and onlookers alike, and certainly causes panic amongst the bystanders when a person has one in a public place. Within the confines of their own home, relatives have often learnt to cope with the occasional attack. The nurse will be involved only if advice is required about the seizure itself or if one occurs in a patient attending the surgery. The principles are simple.

1 Give the patient as much room as possible so that damage by falling on furniture, sharp corners, etc., does not occur. If the nurse is present, she notes the time the seizure begins for later recording.
2 Try and control the body movements gently but not by forcible restraint.
3 If it is possible to get a wedge, such as a mouth gag, tongue depressor or spoon, between the teeth, this will stop the patient biting the tongue, but do not insert fingers or anything which might accidently be swallowed.
4 The convulsion part of the seizure will last only a very short time, and then the patient usually becomes still and comatose or semi-comatose for a varying period of time depending on the severity of the attack. During this period the patient should be moved into the semiprone position and treated as any other unconscious patient.
5 When consciousness has been regained and the patient is talking coherently he or she can be allowed to go home with a friend or relative after verifying some details for the nurse.
6 The nurse checks whether the patient is taking medication regularly, and records the seizure in the patient's notes with details of duration, incontinence and other relevant information such as whether the patient's entire body was affected.

Cardiovascular emergencies

Myocardial infarction

Patients with severe angina or a frank myocardial infarct will sometimes arrive in surgery unaware of how ill they are. The classical symptoms are severe, crushing central chest pain with or without radiation into the jaw and left arm. The patient will feel very unwell, pale, faint and sweaty. However, these gross symptoms are not always present and a patient may collapse on the surgery premises without prior warning.

Any history which can be obtained will be valuable and if the patient is already taking medication such as trinitrin sublingually, give the patient a tablet immediately. Check the pulse and blood pressure and seek aid from a doctor at once.

An unconscious patient may have had a cardiac arrest, and if no pulse or blood pressure reading is discernible then immediate cardiac massage and mouth-to-mouth resuscitation should be started. Further drugs may be used at the discretion of the doctor and should be kept on the emergency tray (see Chapter 6).

If an emergency call is received, when no doctor is immediately available for a patient who has collapsed at home with symptoms suggestive of a myocardial infarction, then it is probably best to summon the help of ambulance personnel and continue trying to contact the doctor.

Transient ischaemic attacks (TIA)

In the elderly patient arteriosclerosis will affect the whole of the arterial tree. From time to time this may result in the normal physiological mechanisms for maintaining the blood flow to be slightly delayed; the cerebral circulation is particularly sensitive in this situation. A sudden change in posture, turning of the head quickly or other quick movements may cause the patient to be transiently giddy or even faint but recovery is almost instantaneous. The only treatment required from the nurse is reassurance and encouragement to the patient to try and change positions more slowly but the doctor may feel that further investigations are necessary. The patient may fall without warning but quickly recovers unless injured in the fall.

Cerebrovascular episode (stroke, CVA)

The arteriosclerosis leading to a TIA can, of course, progress to a more major cerebral catastrophe with unconsciousness, hemiparesis or hemiplegia. If it occurs in the surgery the action taken is that for the unconscious patient. If it occurs at home the relatives should be advised to leave the patient wherever he or she has fallen, make the patient as comfortable as possible, remove dentures if applicable, and reassure the relatives that the doctor will visit as quickly as possible.

The presence or absence of medical help immediately is unlikely to make any difference to the outcome. A patient suffering from a massive stroke will die very quickly, but most are not so dramatic and indeed the patient may well have gained consciousness with only minor residual signs of neurological damage when the doctor arrives, or with more overt signs of a hemiparesis or hemiplegia.

Anaphylactic shock

Anaphylactic shock is caused by a major allergic reaction to an injection, usually a densensitising vaccine, or to something more specific such as a penicillin injection. Occasionally it is the result of insect stings. Because it is life-threatening the action to be taken in this emergency must be discussed between the nurse and the doctor, as it is a rare event. If it does occur immediate action is life-saving and there will be no time to consult other medical staff.

The history will be obvious because the patient will collapse within a very short time of receiving the injection or sting. The reaction can sometimes be delayed and it is the risk of anaphylactic reaction which has brought desensitising vaccines into disrepute. Collapse is swift and immediate action is necessary. The treatment is either adrenaline subcutaneously 1/1000 strength 1 ml in an adult or correspondingly less in a child. This can be followed by 100 mg hydrocortisone intramuscularly or intravenously if a doctor is present to give it.

Hypoglycaemic coma

Diabetics on insulin are always at risk of having a hypoglycaemic attack and should be aware of this. Part of the education of a diabetic is to explain about the risks of hypoglycaemia and the patient should be taught the early signs so that action can be taken before unconsciousness supervenes. These episodes in patients on oral hypoglycaemic treatment are usually very mild and infrequent, if at all.

The first sign of an impending hypoglycaemic attack is usually a feeling of faintness and hunger. This quickly passes on to confusion, aggressive behaviour and finally coma. The patient is pale, sweating and restless. The episode occurs when a dose of insulin has been taken and then for whatever the reason, such as being in too much of a hurry to get to work, the dose of insulin is not 'covered' by the appropriate amount of carbohydrate. It will, of course, also occur if the dose of insulin given is too large so that the carbohydrate metabolism is disturbed and the blood sugar falls rapidly or if the patient does not have their usual meal after the insulin.

If the patient is conscious and still cooperative then he or she should be given a drink of orange juice or tea containing several teaspoons of sugar. In this situation one does not worry about exceeding the normal quantity of sugar in the diet as it is imperative to raise the blood sugar levels rapidly to prevent coma. Extra carbohydrate in the form of sugar lumps or biscuits can also be used. When the patient has recovered he or she should have the next meal as usual.

Often the transition from an awareness of symptoms to coma is fairly rapid or else no one else is present to seek help. In this case the patient will be unconscious and a doctor will be required to inject intravenous dextrose or intramuscular glucagon. The hypoglycaemic coma is a true emergency because the longer the patient is unconscious the greater the risk of permanent brain damage from the low blood sugar.

Hyperglycaemic coma

The opposite situation to hypoglycaemia is hyperglycaemia when there is too much sugar in the blood.

The practice nurse will rarely be involved with this situation as it usually develops over a day or so when the diabetic has either stopped taking insulin for some reason or has an intercurrent infection which has disturbed the insulin requirements of the patient. The patient does not go rapidly into a coma as occurs with a low blood sugar and the medical management usually warrants hospital admission for restabilisation.

Trauma

Lacerations

The arrest of haemorrhage is discussed on page 90. Most simple lacerations can be sutured in the treatment room and the materials required for these are described in Chapter 5.

In general all wounds which are gaping, especially on the scalp, fingers or over joint surfaces, will need suturing. Some nurses are trained by the doctor to do simple suturing but this will be left to the individual discretion of the practice. What the nurse must expect to do is assess an injury which she sees in the treatment room so that medical advice can be sought for the appropriate ones.

The introduction of the transparent self-adhesive steristrip has reduced the number of injuries which need suturing. This is particularly useful for children, and on small cuts produces better effects than suturing as there are no stitch marks around the wound. Using steristrip on areas where the strip cannot stick easily or on skin which is repeatedly stretched (e.g. a finger joint), inappropriately, is doomed to failure and it is better to insert a suture or two at the time rather than be left with a gaping wound several days old if steristrip has been used and failed to hold the edges of the cut together.

All patients who have an open wound must have their tetanus state checked from the records and an appropriate course given by the practice nurse if they are not adequately covered.

Burns

The immediate first aid treatment for a burn when possible is to put the affected area into cold water. It is worth mentioning this to patients as cold immersion considerably reduces the area of tissue damage produced by heat.

If redness only has occurred and the area is small then no treatment is required at all. Sunburn is commonly seen as a first or even second degree burn in the treatment room. Soothing creams and calamine lotion are all that are required if blistering has not occurred. In severe sunburn analgesics and antihistamines will also make the patient more comfortable.

When blistering occurs it is best to puncture the blister with a sterile needle and express the serum, otherwise the blister will usually burst or be rubbed off anyway, leaving an exposed raw area. If the burnt area is extensive then it may be necessary to put a sterile dressing on it, but smaller areas are better left exposed to the air.

Flamazine (silver sulphadiazine 1%) has proved to be very useful in dressing burns. This can be used in conjunction with tulle or a dry dressing.

Sprains

A patient who has suffered a minor injury to a joint may tear or bruise the tissues around the joint producing pain, swelling and localised tenderness. The history usually makes the situation clear and analgesia, support for the joint and gentle mobilisation is the treatment. Severely sprained large joints such as the ankle will need strapping with Elastoplast (elastic adhesive plaster) rather than a crepe bandage. If using Elastoplast first protect the skin with gauze or kling bandage before applying it.

Fractures

The majority of patients who have an obvious fracture will be transported directly to an accident and emergency department. However, minor fractures will be presented in the treatment room, usually associated with other trauma such as bruises, sprains or lacerations.

Small flake fractures associated with severe sprain of a joint, especially the ankle, can be treated as for a sprain unless the pain and swelling are too severe, when a plaster of Paris support will have to be applied for two or three weeks.

Some isolated practices may do much more in the way of dealing with trauma, but it is felt beyond the scope of this book to go into the details of setting fractures or other major casualty work.

REFERENCES

1   Skeet M. (1981) *Emergency Procedures and First Aid for Nurses*. Blackwell Scientific Publications.

Chapter 9

Simple Medical Conditions

The workload of general practice is variable because of many factors. The obvious ones are those due to epidemics of common illnesses such as influenza and measles. Other factors governing workload include the attitudes of the doctors and staff to their patients and the efficiency or otherwise of the practice organisation.

THE PRINCIPLES OF SELF-MANAGEMENT

One area which can easily be neglected but is probably the easiest to influence is that of self-management by the patient. Management of simple uncomplicated illnesses which are self-limiting and require no special knowledge or treatment by the patient without recourse to medical advice still reduce the routine workload enormously. There will always be those patients who, because of their inability to cope, attitudes to illness or pressures from other factors such as marital stress, will always need to be supported through the most minor of illnesses. These are a small proportion of the patients in the practice and the majority can be helped to acquire the knowledge to manage simple situations for themselves.

The best time to educate patients on health matters is at the time of the contact with medical personnel. At this time they are highly motivated to learn about their illness and are at their most susceptible to education. Patients retain or recall afterwards very little of what went on in the consultation so the information imparted has to be simple and repeated frequently. To reinforce this learning it is useful to have extra leaflets or other information, to hand the patient as he or she leaves so that it can be read later. The Health Education Council produces many leaflets and booklets on a wide variety of subjects and their local branch will be delighted to supply any practice with a good supply of this material. Unfortunately, a great deal of adverse publicity to commonsense management, such as the use of aspirin, is produced by ill-informed reports in popular journals or on television about scientific papers.

In recent years many more effective remedies such as antidiarrhoeals or decongestants have become available from the chemist without a prescription. Indeed it is often cheaper to buy a medication than have to pay a prescription charge and the nurse should be familiar with this range of preparations to advise patients accordingly. This subject will be considered in more detail in Chapter 12.

Bearing these factors in mind, there are a number of common conditions which may be considered for appropriate self-management.

UPPER RESPIRATORY INFECTIONS

The majority of upper respiratory symptoms due to infection are caused by viruses. As such, they are self-limiting conditions and only require symptomatic treatment to make them more tolerable to the patient. It is only when secondary bacterial infection supervenes that antibiotics may be required (e.g. this is commonly found in sinusitis and some cases of otitis media), thus, instructions to issue to patients may be verbal, written, or a combination of both and include:

1   Reassurance that all is going to settle in the course of a few days
2   The value of analgesia/antipyretic compounds, such as aspirin or paracetamol, in appropriate dosage. Aspirin is not recommended for children under 12 years old
3   A few suggestions about proprietory cough linctuses or decongestants. Remember to warn patients that many of these substances contain antihistamines and may, therefore, cause drowsiness
4   Advice about environment:
    (a)   bed is not necessary unless the patient feels more comfortable there
    (b)   central heating and a crowded, smokey atmosphere is not conducive to helping the symptoms
    (c)   if apyrexial the only value in being away from work is to prevent passing the infection on to other people
5   Self-certification. For all cases of minor illnesses, patients are expected to self-certify themselves away from work on form SC1 for the first six days of sickness. This is usually more than sufficient for most cases of upper respiratory infection and if the symptoms have not resolved at the end of this time the patient should probably be seeking medical advice anyway.

In addition to general instructions such as those listed the nurse should bear in mind that some patients will use minor illness as an 'excuse' to visit the doctor when they really wish to discuss an alternative subject. In this instance, children are sometimes used as the presenting complaint to enable the parent to talk about something quite unrelated. For this reason any patient who seeks medical advice for apparently trivial symptoms should not be denied the opportunity to do so. It is then the responsibility of the doctor or nurse to give the patient an opportunity to ventilate other problems if the consultation seems inappropriate for the symptoms presented. Patients who repeatedly insist on seeking medical advice for minor respiratory illness should be constantly encouraged to start taking some responsibility for their own health and that of their family.

Asthma

The term *asthma* merely means wheezing, but it is an emotive word to the patient or parent, conjuring up visions of being desperately ill and fighting for breath. It is becoming more medically acceptable to use the term for any condition where a wheeze is present, as studies show that a number of patients, particularly children, are far more disabled than they need to be because no one has formally diagnosed them as asthmatic and treated them vigorously.

Many children become a little wheezy with respiratory infections and only require a mild antispasmodic such as salbutamol (Ventolin) to take on these occasions. However, more severe asthmatics will need regular medication which is often abused. It is abused by being taken far too frequently during an acute attack when medical advice should be sought or by using the inhaler ineffectively. In recent years there has been a large influx of inhalers onto the market and it is important that the nurse understands the principles behind the use of these inhalers and how they should be used correctly. The action of the various inhalers is described in Chapter 11.

GASTROINTESTINAL DISORDERS

Diarrhoea and vomiting are common symptoms, particularly amongst children. While most of these episodes are relatively trivial and self-limiting the risk of dehydration in young children or the masking of more severe pathology, such as intestinal obstruction, has always to be borne in mind.

Causes

The causes of diarrhoea and vomiting are many. Age is an important consideration when trying to make a decision about likely cause and future management. It is emphasised that the object of this chapter is not to turn the nurse into a doctor but enable her to have guidelines when consulted by patients with these symptoms. Some of the major causes in order of frequency are:

Vomiting

1 Viral, bacterial or toxic causes in all age groups.
2 Feeding problems in babies.
3 Menierè's disease or labyrinthitis in middle aged and elderly, particularly if there have been previous episodes.
4 Migraine—will be associated with the other classic symptoms.
5 Middle ear or upper respiratory infection in children.
6 Intestinal obstruction, particularly in babies and the elderly.

Diarrhoea

1 Following vomiting, almost always infective and usually viral.
2 On its own at any age, infections, occasionally from contaminated food.
3 Other bowel disorders such as ulcerative colitis. The length of history will usually give the clue to these conditions.
4 Spurious diarrhoea in the elderly is caused by faecal leakage around impacted faeces.

Management

1 In simple uncomplicated cases where the patient is not very young (over one year) and the history is only a matter of hours, then frequent small sips of fluid, starvation until symptoms have subsided and a mild bowel sedative such as kaolin are all that are required.
2 All patients who are advised as in 1 should be told to contact the practice again if symptoms persist for 24 hours or if abdominal pain is persistent or severe.
3 Children under a year old or any patients when the symptoms do not fit into the infective pattern should be referred to the doctor the same day as should any patient in whom symptoms have persisted for more than 24 hours and who are not obviously improving.

EAR INFECTIONS AND EAR SYRINGING

The practice nurse must reinforce her skills with an auriscope to visualise the external meatus of the ear and also the drum itself. She should be familiar with the appearance of the normal drum and when it is appropriate to syringe an ear.

Ear syringing should be done only when wax is clearly the problem and the patient has has no pain or discharge from the ear and there is no history of perforation of the drum or mastoiditis. In all other circumstances she should not syringe an ear without first consulting the doctor. The technique for syringing is described in Chapter 5.

Children in particular are susceptible to middle ear infections following a cold and any child who complains of earache should be examined. If the drums are not absolutely normal then the nurse should refer to the doctor for advice.

Throat infections or erupting teeth will also give referred pain to the ears and so the mouth and throat should also be examined.

The prescribing of antibiotics and other medication for these conditions will obviously depend upon the discretion of the doctor and commonly used preparations are described in Chapter 12.

EYE CONDITIONS

Patients will frequently present to the nurse with painful red eyes and as the range of conditions possible is very great the nurse must treat all of these cases with extreme care. If in any doubt whatsoever the patient must be seen by a doctor.

General principals for examining the eye

1   Get the patient in a good light.
2   Look at the lids and surrounding tissues for abnormality.
3   Check the pupil for the light reflex by shining a torch into the eye and seeing both pupils contract.
4   Look for localised signs of inflammation especially on the conjunctive, the sclera or the lids.

Conjunctivitis

This is a common condition with a variety of causes. The signs are:

1   A painful red eye with inflammation across the conjunctiva making the eye look pink. One or both eyes may be affected.
2   Discharge which may be purulent or just excessive tears.
3   Vision is normal.

The important differential diagnosis for conjunctivitis is to exclude a foreign body from the surface of the eye as all the other causes will probably require a prescription anyway.

Foreign body

1 The history of getting a piece of dust or similar material in the eye will give an important clue.
2 Usually one eye only is affected.
3 A gritty feel or pain is always present.
4 The eye will be red and probably watering but in simple cases there will be no discharge.

When examining the eye for a foreign body the lid should be everted over a matchstick or orange stick to check under the lid. Stand behind the seated patient with their head supported and put the stick longitudinally over the upper eyelid. Gently hold the eyelashes between the fingers of the other hand and pull the lid gently downwards while exerting gently pressure on the lid with the stick. Now flick the lid upwards over the stick and it will evert allowing the underside to be seen. A piece of grit may be found adhering to this and be easily removed with a piece of gauze or cotton wool on a stick. Intense pain may make it difficult to perform this procedure and the nurse should not continue if unable to do it easily as it is a simple manoeuvre in uncomplicated circumstances.

Foreign bodies on the surface of the eye may be seen with a good light, especially if it is angled across the eye striking the cornea at about 45° rather than directly. They can often be removed with cotton wool on an orange stick after anaesthetising the eye using local anaesthetic drops.

If a foreign body is suspected but not seen on examination then the eye should be stained with fluorescein drops which come provided in a sealed individual dose dropper, as do most eye preparations such as anaesthetics or mydriatics. A few drops of fluorescein instilled into the eye and allowed to stain for a few minutes will help to identify foreign bodies, corneal abrasions or dentritic ulcers.

(a) Corneal abrasions occur if a foreign body scratches the cornea but is then washed away by the tears. Scratches also occur on the cornea, often when parents are playing with their children and a fingernail just catches the eye. Fluorescein stains abrasions fluorescent yellow/green where epithelial cells have been removed from the surface of the cornea. They can easily be seen when stained by using a good light as described earlier.

Abrasions need local antibiotic drops (e.g. chloramphenicol) for a few days and the eye needs to be covered or the patient must wear dark glasses and they heal without further problem.

Incidentally, any eye which has had local anaesthetic drops in it must be covered for 4–6 hours until the corneal reflex has recovered in case a further foreign body got in the eye and severely damaged it with the patient being unaware of it. If a foreign body penetrates the cornea the eye should be covered and the patient referred.

(b) Dendritric ulcers. These are caused by a herpes like virus and can produce considerable damage in the eye if unrecognised. The symptoms are often identical to a foreign body, pain and a unilateral red eye. However, when stained the ulcer appears as a tiny branching structure rather like the branches of a tree than the single line or mark of a simple abrasion. If the nurse is in any doubt the patient should be referred for a further opinion.

All other causes of conjunctivitis are usually infective or allergic and will require assessing with appropriate treatment. Very young babies often get conjunctivitis or a purulent discharge from the eye when they get an upper respiratory infection. The reason for this is that the tears and tear duct system are often not fully developed until the baby is about six months old and therefore the normal protective mechanism of the eye is inefficient. One should always bear in mind the rare case of gonococcal conjunctivitis in the new born or very young as this is an extremely serious infection which needs urgent treatment of mother and child.

Other causes of painful eyes

There are many other causes for a painful eye or eyes and the management of these is not in the realm of the practice nurse except to recognise that referral is required.

Acute glaucoma is probably the most significant as it can lead to loss of vision. In this condition the intraocular pressure of the eye rises, the cornea is often hazy, vision is poor and the patient is in pain. This is an emergency as sight is rapidly lost and the patient should be referred for a specialist opinion. Chronic glaucoma is more common but does not usually present acutely. The onset is more insidious, possibly with headaches, but treatment is necessary to prevent loss of vision.

Herpes zoster (shingles) may present as pain in the eye or forehead before the typical eruption starts. Once the vesicles begin to develop the diagnosis is obvious and the patient should be referred for treatment.

SKIN RASHES

There are many causes for rashes on the skin and it is far too complex a problem to be described in detail. The nurse should take every possible opportunity to see rashes presenting in the surgery and to be reminded by the doctor of their cause and salient features. In this way she will soon learn to identify the common infectious diseases of childhood such as measles, and other common infections such as athletes' foot or herpes zoster.

The major features of some common conditions are described but the only way to make a confident diagnosis about rashes is to see good examples of them and then remember what they looked like.

Measles

The child is unwell and has usually been so for several days. He or she is catarrhal with a hard non-productive cough and a temperature of about 39°C (101°F). The eyes are often red and the rash itself is a blotchy, flat rash over the trunk, head and limbs. It often starts behind the ears and will slowly develop over the ensuing 24 hours. Koplik's spots look like tiny white grains of salt on the mucous membrane of the mouth and appear before the rash. They are thus a useful diagnostic pointer in children whose appearance and story is suggestive of measles before the rash has actually appeared.

There is no specific treatment except symptomatically or if secondary infection, such as middle ear inflammation, supervenes several days after the illness first appears. The child is ill for about a week and probably needs to be off school for about two weeks. The incubation period is ten days when advising about contacts or the possibility of siblings acquiring the disease.

Measles vaccine is commonly given at the age of one year, but only offers about 70% protection to children in measles epidemics. However, one can reassure the parents of children who get measles despite vaccination that the illness will run a much milder course than the full blown disease.

Rubella (German Measles)

Rubella is becoming less common since routine immunisation of girls was introduced. Nevertheless there is still a lot of anxiety in parents when their child has a rash and they should be reassured.

The rash of typical rubella is much more diffuse than measles and is often very striking on the face. The diagnosis should not be made if the posterior occipital chain of lymph glands cannot be palpated, as many virus infections produce a transient non-specific rash very similar to rubella. The rubella rash lasts for several days whereas the other imitative virus infections seldom last more than 24 hours. No treatment is required and children only need to be kept out of contact with expectant mothers. It is still necessary for girls to be immunised for rubella even if they are thought to have had the clinical infection because a firm diagnosis is often in doubt.

Chicken pox

The characteristic lesion in chicken pox is a small blister-like spot with clear serous fluid in the centre. There will be many of these scattered over the trunk and face and they will show various stages of development from an early red spot, through the vesicular (blister) stage to crusting and the formation of a scab. The diagnosis will usually be obvious, especially as chicken pox tends to occur in minor outbreaks of cases, and apart from being febrile and irritable the child is not at risk. Treatment with calamine lotion helps to cool down the irritating spots and encourage them to dry and crust over and an antihistamine such as promethazine (phenergan) will reduce the itch and sedate the patient in more severe cases. It helps to put the child in a tepid bath or add sodium bicarbonate to the water to reduce irritation.

OTHER RASHES

Eczema

Infantile

Infantile eczema occurs in babies a few months old in which there is no family history of eczema. Seborrhoeic eczema is found in the scalp (cradle cap) and only needs to be emulsified with olive oil in most cases.

Nappy rash is a form of infantile eczema in which the skin in the nappy area is severely inflamed and excoriated. It is often infected secondarily with monilia (thrush) and may need specific treatment from the doctor. The milder cases can be treated by using barrier creams such as drapolene and keeping the baby out of nappies altogether when lying in the cot.

Atopic eczema appearing in the skin folds or as a dryness on the face can be treated with simple creams such as Nivea, but when more severe requires further advice and responds well to simple dilute hydrocortisone preparations.

Adult

Eczema in adults is either due to a sensitivity reaction to an external cause such as a metal watchstrap or detergent or is the atopic variety when there is usually a history of previous episodes.

Contact eczema is usually obvious, if thought of, as it begins by being localised to the contact area. Frequent sensitivities are metal straps, buckles, medallions, detergents, rubber gloves and certain types of plants such as primula.

Atopic eczema is often severe and needs medical advice if more than a mild dryness and irritation of the skin. It begins in the flexures of the skin, elbows, knees, etc., but can easily spread to be extensive over the trunk and limbs. Systemic antihistamines and topical steroids are the mainstay of treatment.

Herpes

Herpes simplex (*cold sore*)

The common lesion caused by the virus *Herpes simplex* is the cold sore on the lip of someone who has had his or her resistance lowered, usually by an upper respiratory illness. The virus is acquired, often as a child from the parent, and lives in the cells of the mucocutaneous junction of the lips. When resistance is lower the virus proliferates, produces a blistering effect which quickly scabs over to produce the large single lesion associated with this condition. The natural history is that the crust dries off in 7–10 days and heals to recur at a later date.

No treatment really affects the course of the lesion except idoxuridine solution (Herpid) or acyclovir cream (Zovirax). They need to be applied as soon as the eruption begins and every two hours during the day. This is very expensive medication and only of limited value. Dabbing the sore with surgical spirit to encourage it to dry up is effective and certainly more economical.

There has been an increasing number of cases of genital herpes occurring as a sexually transmitted disease. This is a very painful condition found on the genitalia, particularly on the labia, and is caused by the same virus as causes the cold sore on the lips. Treatment in this case would certainly be justified as the condition is very distressing.

Herpes zoster

Herpes zoster is the eruption of vesicles seen along the line of a somatic nerve, commonly one on the trunk. The cause is the re-activation of the chicken pox virus which has lain dormant in the dorsal ganglion of the nerve for many years, therefore a person must have had chicken pox to develop *herpes zoster*.

The lesions run along the line of the cutaneous nerve and therefore have the specific distribution of that nerve. It will be unilateral, stopping at the mid-line, and is characterised by intense pain. Often the pain is the presenting feature before the rash has actually developed and this will follow within a day or so. The vesicles dry up and fade over the course of 10 to 14 days but the pain may persist as post-herpetic neuralgia.

The treatment essentially consists of encouraging the lesions to dry quickly and avoiding secondary infection of them. The pain should be treated with adequate analgesia (usually something stronger than paracetamol is required) as the incidence of post-herpetic neuralgia seems to be reduced in those whose pain was adequately controlled in the early stages of the disease. Topical application of idoxuridine or a acyclovir may also be prescribed.

MUMPS

The child with mumps usually presents with a unilateral or bilateral swelling of the parotid salivary gland which is found in front of the ear and extends down over the angle of the jaw. Large cervical glands are often confused by patients as being mumps, but the diagnosis is simple if one remembers that the salivary gland extends up the side of the face, and therefore this area must be swollen and tender to pressure to confirm the diagnosis. The submandibular salivary glands may also be involved but it is rare for these to be swollen without the parotid ones being involved.

After the first 24–48 hours, when there is general malaise, pyrexia and some pain as the glands swell, the child is not usually very ill. Treatment consists of analgesia, plenty of fluids and careful oral toilet as the mouth becomes very dry without much saliva being produced for several days. The child can return to school between one and two weeks of the onset of the illness when the glands have subsided and the malaise has gone.

Adults who have not had mumps in childhood are at risk of catching it, especially if their children get it. Here the course of illness is usually more severe and occasionally other organs such as the testes, ovaries and pancreas may be affected.

A mumps vaccine is now available and routinely used on the North American continent and is being introduced to the UK (MMR vaccine).

INFESTATIONS OF THE SKIN

Head and body lice

Pediculosis pubis and capitis are seen more commonly now in the general population than they used to be. The infestation of school children has reached epidemic proportions and infestation can occur in even the most scrupulously careful household.

Head lice are usually first noticed as nits. These are the eggs and are laid at the base of the hair close to the scalp. Newly laid eggs will be close to the scalp and those further out and white are hatched eggs which have moved away from the scalp as the hair grows. The louse itself is very small and difficult to see. It passes from one head to another by contact.

Lice on the body are usually found in the pubic hair and are more easily seen than head lice as they are larger, about the size of a pinhead.

The treatment is thorough soaking in one of a number of solutions, but malathion is probably the most effective. Indeed the lice seem to be becoming immune to some of the proprietary preparations and shampoos which can be bought over the counter, such as Prioderm shampoo. After putting on the lotion and leaving it on the hair overnight the patient or parent shampoos the infected hair in the morning. The whole procedure should be repeated a few days later to kill any further lice which have hatched after the first application. All members of the family should be treated, even if they show no signs of infestation, as otherwise it can become difficult to eradicate it from the family as members reinfect each other.

Scabies

Scabies is caused by a small arthropod which burrows just below the surface of the skin and lays its eggs at the end of a tunnel some few millimetres long. It can only be transmitted by close and prolonged contact with an infected person. It causes intense irritation of the skin and the classical burrow lesions can usually be found in the web of the fingers or the wrist. Although these are common sites it must be assumed that the whole skin, except the head, will be infected.

Treatment consists of having a hot bath and scrubbing the affected areas vigorously. After drying, benzyl benzoate lotion or gamma benzene hexachloride is applied with cotton wool from neck to toes, paying particular attention to the skin folds. This is left to dry and 24 hours later a further application applied. After a further 24 hours the whole body can be bathed and that should be the end of the episode. The skin will stay irritable for several days after treatment and partners should also be treated.

INSECT BITES

Insect bites are usually easily diagnosed as the lesions are single and very irritating. Some bites cause a blister to form in the centre of the lesion and in these cases it should be burst with a sterile needle and a dry dressing applied. All other bites are best treated with calamine lotion plus antihistamine tablets (e.g. Piriton) if the irritation is severe.

WASP AND BEE STINGS

Insect stings usually cause pain in the lesion but require little treatment in the majority of cases, except reassurance of the patient. A bee may leave the sting behind and this may be removed by gripping with a pair of forceps and pulled out. If the reaction is severe or the person is known to be allergic to stings then they should immediately commence on a course of antihistamine tablets for a few days. In rare cases of severe allergy, an anaphylactic reaction can occur (see Chapter 8).

There are a number of topical applications available over the counter (e.g. Waspease) but these have limited value except as reassurance.

FOREIGN BODIES

Eye

Foreign bodies in the eye are discussed on page 104.

Nose

Children are remarkably adept at pushing an assortment of items up their noses. A common object is a marble and this can be extremely difficult to remove. The risks of pushing the object further and further up the nose should be borne in mind. If it is small enough to go into the posterior nasal cavity it can then fall down into the posterior pharynx and be inhaled into the airway. Thus foreign bodies in the nose should be approached cautiously and if not easily removed with fine-toothed forceps the patient should be referred to the doctor.

Ear

A similar assortment of items may be found in the external auditory meatus. Cotton wool may have become impacted, a piece of matchstick broken off by someone attempting to dewax their ears, or other objects inserted for one reason or another.

Provided that a good view is obtained through an aural speculum, many of these can be removed with a fine pair of forceps, but if the removal is causing pain or bleeding, then the patient should be referred to the doctor. After removal of the object the drum and meatus should be examined carefully to exclude unexpected damage to them.

REFERENCES

1   Lane D. & Starr A. (1981) *Asthma—the facts*. OUP.
2   Pearson R. (1987) *Asthma Care in General Practice*. Asthma Society Training Centre, Stratford on Avon.

Chapter 10

Contraception

Providing contraceptive counselling and advice to his or her patients is an important service provided by the general practitioner. The volume of this type of work has risen steadily in the last decade and the doctor can be given valuable assistance in this activity by a family planning trained nurse.

Family planning clinics, organised and staffed by local authority employed personnel, have been established for many years and have been a useful source of free advice and help to women. Some patients prefer to attend a family planning clinic rather than their own doctor because they:

(a) Have always sought contraceptive advice at a clinic
(b) Prefer to see a woman doctor if one is not available in the practice
(c) Prefer anonymity
(d) May be too diffident about seeking advice from a doctor whom they may have known since childhood
(e) Do not perceive the role of the GP to include the giving of contraceptive advice.

These are all valid reasons except the last. It is important that the GP not only perceives his or her role to include the giving of contraceptive advice but that his patients are aware of this and of the advantages of attending their own doctor for contraceptive help. The advantages are that:

(a) They will see a doctor who has known them for a long time and will be aware of their background, medical or social
(b) If problems arise with the contraceptive used, these may have to be presented to the GP anyway, and it is better that he or she is aware of the decision about contraceptives and any hormones used
(c) The general practitioner is available every day and not just at clinic times

(d)   Any of the feminine needs for counselling can be met by employing a trained nurse to help with contraceptive work if a woman doctor is not available

(e)   The advice is confidential and impartial. Patients should not be afraid to go to a doctor whom they have known a long time and they should be aware that no divulgence of information to parents or other interested parties would occur without their permission

(f)   If she does not attend a specific clinic session in the practice no one need know why she has seen her doctor

(g)   Contraception and sexually transmitted disease in the young are often associated problems and the practice may be best situated to advise on these.

FAMILY PLANNING TRAINING FOR NURSES

The Family Planning Association runs courses to train nurses in the whole area of giving contraceptive advice and counselling.

The course includes:

(a)   Three or four days of formal teaching and group discussion. This includes the various techniques available, sexually transmitted disease, psychosexual problems, advice on abortion and the menopause

(b)   Attendance at a series of clinics to gain practical experience under the supervision of a trainer

(c)   Completion of the course—theoretical and practical—and the demonstration of ability in this area of expertise results in the awarding of a Family Planning Certificate of Competence.

The English National Board of the United Kingdom Central Council offers separate courses in family planning, venereal and sexually transmitted diseases and psychosexual counselling.

CONTRACEPTIVE ADVICE

When the patient seeks advice about contraception she will usually see the doctor first, but not necessarily so if she is already aware that the nurse is family planning trained and willing to discuss problems with her. Throughout this discussion it will be assumed that the patient is female as men rarely seek this type of advice (the only exception being when couples come together to discuss contraception or sterilisation).

Whether the doctor or the nurse first sees the patient for contraceptive advice it is important that a number of aspects are considered in turn.

Criteria for contraception

Many improvements have been made over the years in contraceptive methods, but still the 'perfect' contraception is yet to be found. Couples are faced with the task of choosing a method suitable for them. The factors when choosing a method are:

1   The safety of the method and any potential health risks
2   The efficiency and reliability of the method
3   The acceptability to both partners
4   The availability—where can it be obtained and how easily is it obtained?
5   The cost—if any.

Choosing a method

Changing age and lifestyle influence trends in contraception. For the younger women where it is important not to get pregnant, the pill is often the first choice, with reliability and convenience as a high priority. During the childbearing years, when it is not disastrous to a family if a child is born, less efficient contraception is often used— condoms are still used by 15% of couples in the 30–40 age group. After couples have completed their families and women return to full-time employment a reliable and efficient contraception is required again. Sterilisation is becoming more popular in the older couples who have completed their family or in those who wish to pursue a career without the complications and ties of family commitments.

Normal menstrual pattern

To assess any abnormal menstrual pattern, the practice nurse must remember the limits of the normal. The normal menstrual pattern for one patient may be abnormal for another, therefore only broad guidelines can be given.

Menstrual periods usually start in a girl at about the age of ten to thirteen years. They are often irregular for the first year or so but normally, around the age of sixteen, the cycle regulates into a regular pattern. The cessation of the menstrual flow usually occurs around the age of forty-five to fifty—the menopause. This can vary considerably, some females becoming irregular with scanty periods for many years before stopping completely, whereas others find that their periods end abruptly.

The menstrual cycle is calculated from the first day of bleeding, called the first day of the cycle. The average normal length of a menstrual cycle is twenty-eight days with an average normal loss over five to six days.

Useful leaflets for young people explaining the start of the menstrual pattern, or for mature women explaining the menopause can be obtained from the Health Education Council or Family Planning Association.

COUNSELLING

The term *counselling* means enabling clients or patients to make their own decisions based on their own needs after being given adequate information, and providing the opportunity to ventilate any fears or anxieties which they may have. This takes time and a practice nurse can be invaluable in helping the doctor to advise the patient in this discussion. It is important not to impose one's own values or judgements when counselling. Areas which will be covered during the discussion include:

The methods available

A   oral contraception
B   intra-uterine devices
C   the cap
D   the condom (or 'sheath')
E   the safe period
F   other methods.

The acceptability of the various methods to the patient

1   The discussion of patient's anxieties or queries
2   Religion and contraception
3   Young people: advice, counselling and risks
4   Methods for older women
5   Administrative aspects
6   The future.

These aspects will now be considered in more detail.

1   THE METHODS

A Oral contraception

There are many combinations of the pill and these can be grouped into three types.
(i)   The combined
(ii)   Progesterone-only
(iii) Triphasic.
The decision on which type of pill the woman will use is taken by the doctor after discussion with the patient.

(i) *The combined oral contraceptive pills* act by inhibiting ovulation.
The advantages of the combined oestrogen/progesterone pill are:
(a)   It is totally reliable if taken as directed.
(b)   It tends to give good menstrual cycle control.
(c)   It is acceptable to patients who have an aversion to the mechanical methods.
The disadvantages are:
(a)   The oestrogen component may increase the risk of thromboembolism, especially in patients who have had previous episodes such as deep vein thrombosis. For this reason it is not advised for women after their mid-thirties.
(b)   It can cause amenorrhoea both during and after ceasing the pill.
(c)   Other side-effects, such as headache or weight gain, may make it unacceptable.
(d)   It may impair glucose tolerance.

(ii) *The progesterone-only pills* act by changing the nature of the endometrium, rendering it less likely to implant the ovum and by change in the cervical mucus making it more hostile to spermatozoa.
The advantages of the progesterone-only pill are:

(a)   It does not have the thrombotic complications.
(b)   It can be taken while the patient is breast feeding.
(c)   It is useful for the older woman (over 34).
The disadvantages are:
(a)   It has a small contraceptive failure rate—about the same as the mechanical methods (4%).
(b)   It does not produce good cycle control and irregular bleeding may occur.
(c)   The side-effects may make it unacceptable.

(iii) *Triphasic pills* act by varying the hormone levels during the cycle. They mimic the normal pattern and give rise to a more normal looking endometrium.
The advantages of the triphasic pill are:
(a)   Give better bleeding pattern.
(b)   Mimic normal cycle pattern and endometrium.
The disadvantages are:
(a)   Increased number of pill taking errors.
(b)   Premenstrual syndrome during third week of cycle.

Post coital contraception using the pill (The 'morning after' pill)

If a woman presents within 72 hours of unprotected intercourse it is often possible to prevent implantation of the ovum by giving two tablets of a combined preparation containing 50 mg of oestrogen (e.g. PC_4 to be repeated after 12 hours. Four tablets are taken in all).

This method can work in two ways, either by preventing implantation or by delaying ovulation. The failure rate is about 4%. Nausea is a common side effect with occasional vomiting. If vomiting occurs within 3 hours a further 2 tablets should be taken.

Oral contraceptive routines

Each practice should agree its routine guidelines to be followed when dealing with patients needing oral contraceptives. These routines can be grouped into two categories:

1   Patients starting the pill for the first time.
2   Routine follow-up for patients already on the pill.

1   Patients starting the pill for the first time

(a)   Consultation with the general practitioner who explains the method fully.
(b)   The practice nurse explains the routine of the full examination and performs checks which include: weight, blood pressure, urine test for albumen and sugar, breast examination (see Chapter 11) and rubella antibodies (5 ml clotted blood).
(c)   Prepare the patient on a couch for pelvic bimanual examination and a cervical smear. She should be undressed below the waist and covered with a blanket. These examinations are usually performed by the doctor. The practice nurse is responsible for preparing the patient and the equipment required for smear and examination and to act as chaperone. Practice nurses are commonly trained to take routine cervical smears but a maximum five-yearly pelvic examination by the doctor should be included in the routine surveillance.
     The equipment required:
     Cuscos vaginal speculum
     KY Jelly
     Disposable gloves
     Container with industrial methylated spirit for fixing slide
     Wooden cervical spatula
     Frosted ended slide and pencil
     Anglepoise light
     Appropriate cervical smear forms and patient instruction leaflet

After the smear and examination are completed a suggested routine is that the patient is given a prescription for three months of the pill and told to return before completing the third pack of pills. The practice nurse instructs the patient on the routine of taking the oral contraceptive for the first pack as follows:

Counting the first day of the period as day one, take the first pill on day one, take one pill daily for twenty-one days (a good time to take the pill is just before retiring to bed at a regular time). Then stop taking the pill for seven days, during which time it is usual to have a period. At the end of the seven days, on day eight, begin the next course of pills, each course of pills beginning on the same day of the week.

Alternatively the patient can take the first pill on day five of her cycle. If this routine is followed other added contraceptive measures must be used (e.g. sheath) for the first two weeks of taking the pill.

If a pill is forgotten at night, it can be taken the next morning, and if vomiting occurs within an hour or so of taking the pill another one should be taken. Minimal side effects may be experienced by some patients, including nausea, breast tenderness, breakthrough bleeding, slight weight gain, headache and amenorrhoea. Most side effects are corrected within the second cycle of taking the pill. Young patients and women under thirty five years of age who are given oral contraceptives are assured of the very small risk of taking the pill.

Practices may wish to design their own patient instruction leaflet and an example is shown in Appendix II.

2 *Routine follow-up for patients already on the pill*

At three months. The patient returns to the practice nurse who checks that the pill is being correctly taken and asks about any worries or possible side-effects. She then checks the weight to note any marked increase, urine for glucose, blood pressure for any significant rise and breasts for lumps. If the patient and practice nurse are both satisfied that the method of contraception is acceptable a further nine month prescription for the pill is prescribed.

Annual checks. At the annual check the practice nurse follows the same routine as at the three month check. A further prescription is given for twelve months supply of the pill.

Alternate years. The routine for this is the same as the annual check plus a cervical smear and bimanual examination of the pelvis undertaken by the GP. Then again a further twelve month supply of the pill is given.

The outline above is only one suggested routine. Practices will vary slightly, for example, in how frequently a cervical smear is taken, but the basic pattern is the same.

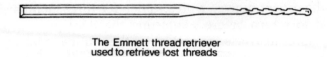

The Emmett thread retriever
used to retrieve lost threads

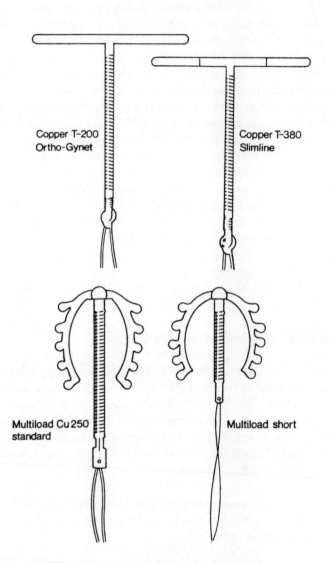

Fig. 10.1   IUCD most commonly used in general practice.

B   The intra-uterine contraceptive device (IUCD)

The modern IUCD containing copper offers a high level of contraceptive reliability. The method involves the insertion in the uterus of a

small plastic and copper device which prevents establishment of the ovum in the endometrium. The copper IUCD devices exert a foreign body reaction which leads to changes in endometrial enzymes and hormone receptors.

New copper bearing devices are being produced (e.g. hormone releasing) as others are being withdrawn from the market. Such devices as Gravigard, Mini-Gravigard and lippes loop are being withdrawn for a variety of reasons and should be replaced with a more modern IUCD when appropriate.

The most commonly used copper bearing devices are shown in Fig. 10.1. The IUCD is more suitable for multiparous women, although the mini copper IUCD can be used in most circumstances for nulliparous women. The indications for using an IUCD are for women who find other methods of family planning are contraindicated or ineffective.

Contraindications for insertion of an IUCD

1 Pelvic inflammatory disease
2 Menorrhagia
3 Pregnancy
4 Fibroids.

Complications and side-effects

1 Pain. This may be experienced, but is usually controlled by mild analgesia. In a few instances severe cramp-like pain persists which may necessitate removing the IUCD.
2 Bleeding. Most women experience vaginal bleeding for a few days after insertion of an IUCD. In some patients the menstrual period can be slightly heavier and longer than normally experienced. Usually after six months the menstrual pattern returns to the patient's normal cycle and loss.
3 Vaginal discharge and pelvic infection.
4 Expulsion.
5 Pregnancy and ectopic pregnancy.

The IUCD is fitted by the GP; the practice nurse's responsibility and role is to prepare and look after the patient and to prepare the equipment for the fitting.

Preparing the patient for IUCD fitting

1 Reassure the patient.

2   Ask the patient to empty her bladder.
3   She should undress from the waist downwards and be covered
     with a blanket.
4   She should then lie on the couch in the lithotomy position.

Equipment and instruments for IUCD fitting (see Fig. 10.2)

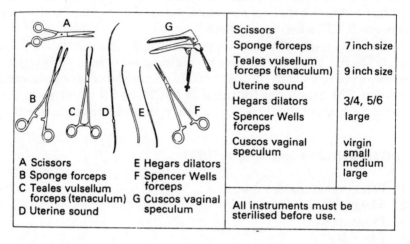

Scissors	
Sponge forceps	7 inch size
Teales vulsellum forceps (tenaculum)	9 inch size
Uterine sound	
Hegars dilators	3/4, 5/6
Spencer Wells forceps	large
Cuscos vaginal speculum	virgin small medium large
All instruments must be sterilised before use.	

A Scissors
B Sponge forceps
C Teales vulsellum forceps (tenaculum)
D Uterine sound
E Hegars dilators
F Spencer Wells forceps
G Cuscos vaginal speculum

Fig. 10.2   Equipment and instruments for fitting an IUCD.

The instruments and equipment are sterilised by boiling or autoclaving and are set out on a trolley with sterile dressing sheets. They include:

Disposable sterile gloves
Cuscos vaginal speculum
Two receivers
Gallipot with savlodil
Sponge holder
Teales vulsellum forceps
Long Spencer Wells forceps
Uterine sound
Hegars uterine dilators, size 3/4 × 2
                                              5/6 × 1
Long curved uterine scissors
KY Jelly
Resuscitation equipment
   —Brook Airway
Cotton wool swabs

Method of inserting an IUCD

During the fitting of the IUCD the role of the practice nurse is to make the patient as relaxed as possible. Often this can be done by explaining to the patient the routine of examination and what to expect during the IUCD fitting. To do this the practice nurse must understand the routine and the role of the GP.

1 First a bimanual examination is carried out to determine the size, shape and position of the uterus and cervix and to eliminate any pelvic abnormalities.
2 A vaginal speculum is then inserted and the cervix and vagina cleansed.
3 Size 3, 4 and 5 uterine dilators are inserted to gradually dilate the cervix.
4 A uterine sound is inserted to determine the length and direction of the uterine cavity.
5 In some instances the vulsellum forceps may be needed to hold the cervix steady.
6 The device is then loaded into the introducer and inserted through the cervical canal.
7 The introducer is then withdrawn.
8 Finally the threads are shortened.

After the completion of the fitting, which usually takes about ten minutes, the patient can be allowed to rest for a while. During this time the practice nurse reassures the patient by explaining that the discomfort the patient may now be experiencing, which is similar to dysmenorrhoea, will be reduced with analgesia. Pain or discomfort is sometimes experienced immediately after fitting because the uterus is attempting to expel the IUCD, causing a colicky pain. The discomfort usually improves after a short time when the patient can then be allowed to go home. During the time the patient is resting the practice nurse explains the method of feeling for the thread of the IUCD. This is done by inserting the index finger into the vagina, where, at the top end of the vaginal wall, the cervix can usually be felt like the tip of a nose. Coming out from the neck of the cervix is the nylon thread of the IUCD which is about 5 cm long. If the patient can feel the thread each month after menstruation it gives her added confidence that the IUCD is in place and has not been expelled during the last menstrual period.

The patient returns to the GP and practice nurse after three months and at this consultation the nurse prepares the patient so that the IUCD can be checked for its position and a record is made of the menstrual flow. If satisfactory, a routine IUCD check is repeated when the loop has been in position for one year and further checks repeated annually. IUCD devices which have copper incorporated into them are removed and replaced three yearly. Some devices can be left in/or up to five years.

The IUCD can be used for postcoital contraception, it helps to prevent implantation of the fertilized ovum, and can be effective up to five days after ovulation. This method may be used for victims of rape.

C   The cap

The cap most commonly used in general practice is the diaphragm dutch cap (see Fig. 10.3a). This cap is made of thin rubber with a firm rim around the edge, in varying sizes to fit comfortably into the vagina. Other caps which can be used are the cervical cap (see Fig. 10.3b), Vault or Dumas cap (see Fig. 10.3c) or Vimule cap which is a combination of the cervical and Vault caps (see Fig. 10.3d).

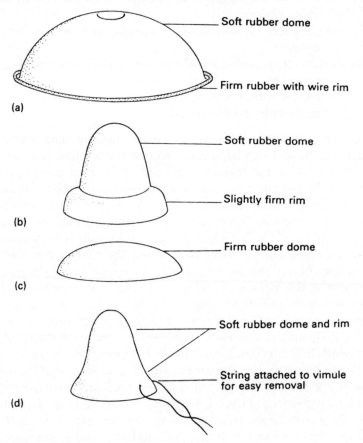

Fig. 10.3   (a) Diaphragm dutch cap. (b) Cervical cap. (c) Dumas cap. (d) Vimule cap.

The cap is placed into position at a suitable time before intercourse and left for six hours afterwards. This method can be used as a satisfactory long term contraceptive for patients waiting to start oral contraceptives or waiting for an IUCD to be fitted. The patient must be highly motivated and encouraged to use the cap regularly with correct creams as described later in the chapter. It can be fitted by the GP or a trained nurse.

At the first visit the patient is fitted with the correct size cap. The cap should fit across the vault of the vagina from the posterior fornix to the retro-pubic space making sure it covers the cervix (see Fig. 10.4). The correct size will fit comfortably and the patient should be unaware of the presence of the cap when in position. The patient should be allowed to feel the cap in the correct position and then told to remove it. Full instructions are then given on the method of inserting the cap herself.

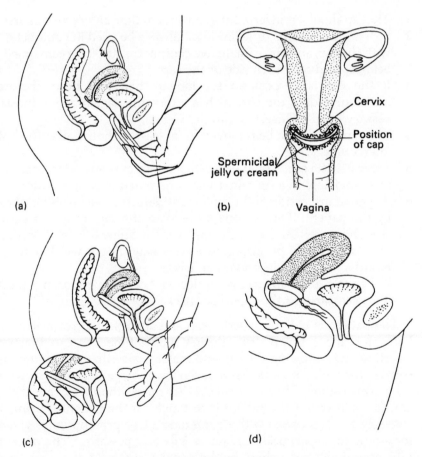

(a) (b)

Cervix

Position of cap

Spermicidal jelly or cream

Vagina

(c) (d)

Fig. 10.4 Insertion and correct position of the cap.

Instructions for the patient

1 Put the cap on the non-dominant hand with the dome uppermost.
2 Pinch rim and hold cap firmly between first finger and thumb of the dominant hand.
3 With non-dominant hand open lips of vulva and insert the cap halfway into the vagina.
4 Tilt the cap upwards slightly.
5 Slide it into the vagina; it should then be in the correct position.
6 Feel for the cervix (it feels like the tip of the nose) through the rubber of the cap.

The patient should be allowed to insert and remove the cap two or three times until she is confident, the nurse checking each time that the position is correct.

Other points to emphasise are:

1 The cap should be inserted at a convenient time before intercourse.
2 Spermicidal creams or jellies must always be used in conjunction with the cap, an approximate five centimetre strip of cream or jelly being spread over each side of the cap.
3 If the cap is in position for longer than two hours before intercourse or if the patient has intercourse again a spermicidal pessary must be inserted into the vagina.
4 The cap should not be removed for at least six hours after the last intercourse.
5 After use the cap should be washed in warm soapy water, rinsed, dried and kept in a container with unscented dusting powder.
6 A regular inspection of the cap for any defects must be undertaken by the patient. This is done by holding the cap up to the light, stretching each section of the cap over the fingers. A small section at a time should be inspected in this way. A cap will last for 6 months to a year, depending on usage.
7 If the patient has an increase or decrease of nine pounds in weight it is necessary for the cap to be checked for a size change.

The patient is given a practice cap and spermicidal cream to take home for about seven days, during which time she can practice inserting and removing the cap and making sure that the method is suitable for both partners. After seven days the patient returns with the cap in position. The nurse checks that the position is correct. If the position is incorrect the patient is re-taught. If the patient is using it correctly and is satisfied with the method a free prescription is given for a new cap, spermicidal cream or jelly and pessaries. The patient returns annually for a check by the practice nurse.

D The condom

The condom or 'sheath' is still a widely used form of contraception and many couples use it satisfactorily. The condom is a sheath made of fine rubber and is disposable after use. It should always be used in conjunction with contraceptive creams, jellies, pessaries or foam which the woman must insert into the vagina before intercourse as an added precaution, in case the sheath splits or comes off. It can only be placed on the erect penis, and the sheath should be unrolled onto the hard erect penis, leaving the last 2 cm or the teat at the blind end of the sheath empty beyond the tip of the penis, allowing room for collection of semen. It must be put on before penetration and removed carefully after withdrawing from the vagina without spilling semen.

The sheath is not available on prescription, but can be purchased from chemist shops, vending machines and other sources, so is a readily available method for couples who have not discussed contraception with their doctor, or prefer not to become involved with the medical profession over an activity which they consider to be private and personal. Sheaths are available free of charge from Family Planning clinics.

The increased risk of HIV infection (AIDS) or other sexually transmitted disease amongst those having multiple partners is reduced by using a condom. This should be encouraged in thoses cases at risk even if another form of contraception (oral or IUCD) is also being used.

E The safe period

(i) *The calendar method*

The principle of the safe period is that fertilisation can occur from two days before to one day after ovulation, therefore the date of ovulation must be calculated exactly. Ideally, the past twelve month cycle should be recorded, noting the first day of bleeding in each cycle. The calculation of the safe period is made by deducting eighteen from the shortest cycle and eleven from the longest cycle (e.g. if a woman's cycle varies from 25 to 31 days):

$$25 - 18 = 7$$
$$31 - 11 = 20$$

The safe period would be days 1–6 and from the 21st day onwards until 6 days after the first day of the next period.

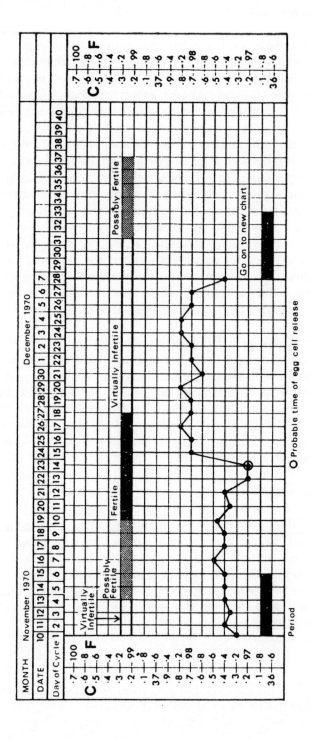

Fig. 10.5 Specimen chart of a 28-day cycle showing (top) time when conception is most likely, and (bottom) an example of temperature variation at different times of the month.

(ii) The temperature method

At ovulation there is a small rise in body temperature (about 0.5°C). If intercourse occurs more than 72 hours after this temperature rise then conception is unlikely in that cycle.

Patients using this method must be highly motivated to take and record their temperature every morning. A special thermometer and chart designed for use for this method of contraception can be purchased from a chemist (see Fig. 10.5). The temperature is taken and recorded on the first day of the cycle, before getting out of bed in the morning and before eating or drinking. The temperature record may vary from day to day but the greatest change is about fourteen days before the next period is due to begin, the approximate day of ovulation. At this time the temperature drops slightly and then rises to the higher level at which it remains until the next menstrual period starts.

The safe period is not reliable and should only be used by those couples in which other methods are unacceptable (e.g. for religious reasons).

F   Other methods

Creams, pessaries, jellies and foams

These are chemical spermicidal agents inserted into the vagina. They should be used in conjunction with a 'sheath' or cap as they do not offer adequate contraceptive protection on their own. Some patients develop allergies to the common preparations and there are some non-allergic preparations on the market. All these agents can be prescribed in the normal way by the doctor with an explanation of their limitations.

The sponge

The sponge is a fairly recently developed barrier method and is placed in the vaginal vault, covering the cervix. It is impregnated with spermicide and can remain in the vagina for 24 hours. The sponge is less effective than the cap and spermicide, but may be convenient for the menopausal woman who does not need a high level of protection.

Coitus interruptus

The withdrawal of the penis from the vagina immediately before ejaculation is called coitus interruptus. Its only advantage is that it does not require the purchase of sheaths or obtaining of contraceptive help before sexual intercourse.

Its disadvantages are that it is highly unreliable and it is easy for the man to forget to withdraw in time, or he can have a premature ejaculation (even if ejaculation occurs at the introitus it is possible for conception to occur). Psychological consequences may arise in both partners from prolonged use of this method. The woman may be constantly anxious about becoming pregnant while using an unreliable method and either or both partners may be left frustrated by interruption of the normal act of intercourse. It may contribute towards frigidity and failure of orgasm for the female partner or impotence in the male. It should only be mentioned to be dismissed in the course of giving contraceptive advice.

Injectable progestogens

The most commonly used injectable progestogen is Depo-Provera, 150 mg given every 12 weeks. This is normally given in the first five days of the cycle. If the woman is postpartum Depo-Provera can be administered five weeks after delivery, and can also be injected within five days of a miscarriage or abortion.

The advantages are:

(a) The injectable progestogens method is highly effective and can reduce menstrual symptoms such as dysmenorrhoea or menorrhagia.
(b) The method is reversible although it may take up to six months for fertility to return.

The disadvantages are:

(a) Once the dose is given the hormone cannot be removed so this means side effects must be tolerated for up to 12 weeks.
(b) With repeated injections patients tend to become amenorrhoeic, with often a delay of return to fertility.
(c) Patients often report weight gain.

2   THE ACCEPTABILITY OF THE METHOD TO THE PATIENT

To make a contraceptive method successful it must be acceptable to both partners. The couple must understand the advantages, disadvantages and techniques of each method so that it is the patient who finally decides on the preferred method. When possible the male partner should be encouraged to participate in the discussion of acceptability. It must be remembered that any method is better than none, so a patient must have freedom of choice.

3 DISCUSSION OF PATIENT'S ANXIETIES OR QUERIES

Most fears of contraceptive methods arise from not understanding the method or the techniques involved. These fears can be overcome by a sympathetic and understanding GP and nurse giving a full explanation. They must gain the patient's complete confidence so that any fears which may arise can be discussed freely. The types of fears which commonly arise during discussion may be: How does an oral contraceptive or IUCD work? How safe is a certain method? Many fears are minor and often unfounded but they must be discussed and answered.

4 RELIGION AND CONTRACEPTION

Religious beliefs may preclude any form of artificial contraception, especially oral or IUCD. The only method of contraception permitted in these circumstances is the safe period.

5 YOUNG PEOPLE: ADVICE, COUNSELLING AND RISKS

Young patients over the age of sixteen are regarded legally as adults and appropriate contraceptive services can be given when requested or needed by these patients. Patients under the age of sixteen who are at risk of having an unwanted pregnancy can, at the GP's discretion, be given contraceptive advice (see below).

Young people who request advice and counselling on contraception must be handled sympathetically and firmly. Advice should be offered about relationships and having intercourse at a young age, the types of contraceptive which may be suitable and appropriate should be discussed. Advice may be given on the dangers of sexually transmitted diseases if this seems appropriate. Although parents should not be informed without the patient's consent, every encouragement should be given to the patient to discuss the whole matter with her mother. It should not be forgotten that in law it is illegal to have intercourse under the age of 16.

6 METHODS FOR OLDER WOMEN

The term *older woman* used in contraception usually means women over the age of 34. In many instances women of this age have completed child bearing. It is medically advisable for these women to be taken off oral contraceptives as the side-effects and complications increase as patients get older. Alternative methods of contraception can be offered, such as the IUCD, cap, sheath, pessaries or sterilisation.

At all times when counselling patients on contraceptive methods the GP and practice nurse should give confidence, encouragement and complete confidentiality.

7   ADMINISTRATIVE ASPECTS

The acceptance of responsibility by the doctor for giving contraceptive advice to his or her patient implies that responsibility is also accepted for supervising the regular routine surveillance of the patient. This means that the patient's record must show what method is being used and when the next check is due. Some practices use a contraceptive card as an insert into the notes and a recall system is vital (Chapter 2).

The practice must decide what is an appropriate period of time between each check and the suggestions in this chapter are those used in only one practice. Nevertheless, it is easy to fall into a time consuming routine which is unnecessary and imposes embarrassing examinations on the patient without evidence that this produces better care. Thus each practice must examine the evidence and decide on a balance between obsessiveness and negligence.

The GP is entitled to claim certain fees from the Family Practitioner Committee for providing contraceptive services, and it is the nurse's responsibility to see that the appropriate forms are available for completion when the patient attends for her check.

Form FP1001

This is completed annually by all patients who have been offered contraceptive advice and/or services from the GP. Even the discussion of various methods and advice about the sheath or safe period qualify, although the patient may not be given a prescription. Of course those who are using methods which do not require regular supervision will not return annually, so it may be that the FP1001 is completed only once for these patients.

Form FP1002

This is used for the fitting of an IUCD. Thereafter an annual fee is claimed on FP1001 for the annual IUCD check. An FP1002 fee can only be claimed once per year even if the IUCD is refitted more than once during the year.

Form FP1003

This is used for temporary residents who have contraceptive advice.

Form FP74

This is used when claiming a fee for taking a cervical smear. A GP may take a smear whenever he feels it is indicated, but he will only be paid for this if:

(a) the patient is over 35 and it is at least five years since her last smear. The first smear after age 35 qualifies and then at 5 yearly intervals
(b) at any age if she has had three pregnancies (including abortions) and it is at least five years since the last smear.

Leaflets

Most contraceptive patient information leaflets and advice literature are available for use in general practice from local Family Planning Clinics or Health Education Councils.

TERMINATION OF PREGNANCY

It is vital that a woman does not enter a sexual relationship with the attitude that 'if anything goes wrong I can always have a termination'. Apart from the undesirability of using termination as a form of contraception there are other risks which include:

(a) A higher incidence of pelvic inflammatory disease.
(b) Cervical incompetence in future wanted pregnancies.
(c) The usual operative risks of anaesthesia and haemorrhage.
(d) The psychological consequences. These have tended to be over-rated by those who do not wish to advise a termination. Evidence suggests that those women who really want a termination feel only relief afterwards and the problems arise in those who are forced into a termination due to circumstances such as being unmarried or already having a large family.

The decision of a doctor to refer a patient for termination of pregnancy will depend on a number of factors which can only be taken into account after careful discussion and counselling with her and preferably her partner. Factors to be considered include the patient's attitude to the pregnancy, past obstetric and contraceptive history, previous terminations, psychiatric or medical history and the duration of the present pregnancy.

The law requires that a statement be completed by two doctors (preferably the GP and the gynaecologist) who have to state that the patient falls into one of the following four categories:

1   The continuation of the pregnancy would involve risk to the life of the pregnant woman greater than if the pregnancy was terminated
2   The continuance of the pregnancy would involve risk of injury to the physical or mental health of the pregnant woman greater than if the pregnancy were terminated
3   The continuance of the pregnancy would involve risk of injury to the physical or mental health of the existing child(ren) of the family of the pregnant woman greater than if the pregnancy were terminated
4   There is substantial risk that if the child were born it would suffer from such physical or mental abnormalities as to be severely handicapped.

The termination itself may be performed within the NHS or privately, but in either case the patient is not likely to be in hospital more than 24 hours if the duration of the pregnancy is less than 12 weeks. Prostaglandin terminations for more advanced pregnancies are less common and require careful decisions on the part of the doctors and patient as to whether the termination of the pregnancy is more desirable than letting it continue.

The moral and ethical aspects of termination have not been considered because each reader will have his or her own opinion on these. Suffice it to say that it is a very emotive subject, but each unwanted pregnancy must be looked upon as a failure of contraception, and in this respect the doctor and nurse must accept some responsibility, particularly if his or her advice was sought beforehand.

All patients who do have a termination must be seen shortly afterwards to discuss contraception and to encourage them to use an efficient method in future.

STERILISATION

Sterilisation is the ultimate contraception but should only be regarded as permanent. Couples increasingly seek advice about sterilisation once they feel they have completed their family and part of contraceptive counselling for older women should include a discussion of the reasons for and against sterilisation for her or her partner.

There are factors to consider before sterilisation.

1   The age of the couple. Surgeons may be reluctant to sterilise a partner if the couple are under 30 years of age.
2   The number of children already produced. Some couples may be adamant that they do not wish to have any children and this wish should be respected once the doctor is convinced that it is the wish of *both* partners.
3   The timing of the request. It is not normally appropriate to take a request for sterilisation too seriously immediately after the birth of a child. However, elective sterilisation may be performed at Caesarean section or after termination of pregnancy if the issue has been discussed and agreed previously.
4   Failure of other methods of contraception or unacceptable side-effects of them.
5   The medical and psychiatric history of the couple.
6   The stability of the relationship.
7   Although the preceding factors have assumed that a couple are requesting sterilisation, it may be only one person. He or she may not have a regular partner but if genuinely seeking sterilisation for good reasons this should not preclude the individual from the opportunity to have the operation.

VASECTOMY

The operation for the male vasectomy entails the cutting of the spermatic cord just as it enters the inguinal canal after leaving the scrotum. It is a simple operation which can easily be performed under local anaesthetic, and which enables the patient to leave the treatment room or hospital quickly after the procedure is completed, although he should not undertake strenuous physical activity for a few days to reduce the possibility of bruising around the operation site.

When discussing this method of sterilisation the following points should be emphasised to the patient:

(a)   It is permanent but not until two consecutive sperm counts are negative.
(b)   It is a simple operation usually done under local anaesthetic.
(c)   There will be no effect on sexual performance including erection and ejaculation.
(d)   As the majority of the ejaculate is made up of secretions from the prostate and other glands entering the urethra, the patient will notice little change in his ejaculate after the operation.

The most reassuring aspect is for the man to know a friend or colleague who has had the operation and is pleased with the result. After the operation the man cannot consider himself infertile until he has had two negative sperm counts. Semen samples are collected monthly from three or four months after the operation until two consecutive sperm counts have revealed no sperm in the ejaculate. Until then contraceptive precautions must be continued.

FEMALE STERILISATION

The female is sterilised as a hospital inpatient by cutting or destroying the fallopian tubes so that the ovum cannot pass down them into the uterus. This may be done by formal abdominal operation such as at Caesarean section, or if there are so many intra-abdominal adhesions that the laparoscopic method is unreliable. The vast majority of female sterilisations are, however, carried out using the laparoscope. This involves making two small (1 cm) incisions in the abdominal wall, one of them being at the umbilicus and the other about halfway towards the symphysis pubis. The laparoscope is inserted through one incision and the cautery equipment through the other. Air is introduced into the peritoneal cavity with the patient tipped slightly head down and this, together with gravity, causes the abdominal organs to fall away exposing the pelvic viscera. The fallopian tubes should be clearly seen through the laparoscope and can then be obliterated by cauterisation or by slipping an elastic band over a fold of tube. This latter method is sometimes used if there is the slightest chance of a reversal of sterilisation being requested at a later date.

The operation has to be performed under general anaesthetic so the patient normally stays in hospital overnight. Within a week the patient is usually fully recovered from any after effects of the operation (faintness, nausea, abdominal discomfort) and, of course, is immediately sterile, unlike the situation in the male. Some gynaecologists prefer to do a hysterogram (X-ray) post-operatively to check that the operation has been successful before allowing unprotected intercourse. The two or three abdominal sutures closing the two small wounds can be removed by the practice nurse a week after the operation. Sexual intercourse can commence within a week or so and no further contraceptive precaution is required. The normal menstrual pattern should be unaffected although there have been suggestions that women who have been sterilised are more likely to have menstrual irregularities as they approach the menopause.

FUTURE TRENDS IN CONTRACEPTION

Many new hormonal and vaccine advances will be available over the next decade, particularly advances in oral contraceptives, injectables or subdermal implants.

Barrier methods will be more widely used since the fear of AIDS. New methods on trial such as a vaginal shield and a disposable loose sheath which covers the whole vagina and external female genitalia may be successful.

FURTHER READING

Guilleland J. (1985) *Contraception. Your questions answered.* Churchill Livingstone.
Guilleband J. (1987) *The Pill.* 3rd edition, OUP.

Chapter 11

Special Clinics

Most practices have special clinics for one purpose or another. The advantage of having clinics is primarily so that one particular problem or condition can be dealt with in a structured fashion on a limited number of patients.

It is easier to have an antenatal clinic where the midwife is present and a routine of weighing, urine testing and examination can be established, rather than having to break off and do these routine tests on a pregnant woman turning up in the ordinary surgery.

Clinics can be divided into three types (Groups 1 to 3 in this chapter).

1 Those where patients are coming for essentially physiological reasons (e.g. antenatal or family planning clinics).
2 Those where the patients suffer from a specific illness (e.g. diabetic or hypertensive clinics).
3 Those where group support and repeated encouragement is required to maintain an activity promoting a healthier existence (e.g. weight reduction or stopping smoking).

The examples discussed are not necessarily all the types of special clinics which can be undertaken. Some practices will have no special clinics, others will have only one or two. One disadvantage of clinics is that everyone attending will know why the other patients are there. This may be particularly embarrassing (e.g. in family planning clinics) and for this reason some patients will prefer the anonymity of an ordinary consultation by appointment—this should not be denied them. The other major disadvantage is that if clinics become large (e.g. antenatal) then there is a risk of the patients being processed; the object becomes one of trying to get the maximum number of patients through in the minimum amount of time rather than allowing enough time for doctor/nurse–patient interaction.

GROUP (1) CLINICS

Antenatal clinics

Although an attached practice midwife will take responsibility for the routine care of the pregnant patient, the practice nurse may sometimes be involved in preparing the patient for examination (e.g. by taking the blood pressure or preparing the patient on the examination couch). The patient attends for the first antenatal visit when she is approximately twelve weeks pregnant. At the first visit a full medical and obstetric history is taken and summarised on a cooperation obstetric record card; this is usually undertaken by the attached midwife but in some circumstances the practice nurse may be involved in doing this. The record card is retained by the patient and brought for all antenatal and postnatal attendances throughout the pregnancy whether at surgery or hospital. The history taken includes both social and medical details.

1 Relevant family history:
   High blood pressure
   Tuberculosis
   Twins
   Diabetes
2 Illness, hereditary disorders and conditions relating to the patient:
   Past medical history
   Epilepsy
   Asthma
   Allergies
   Blood transfusions given in past
   Drug therapy
   Any specific drugs taken in the first three months of pregnancy
3 Social history:
   Smoking and alcohol consumption
   Marital status
   Social conditions at home.

At the first antenatal visit the nurse prepares the patient for a full examination by the general practitioner which includes examination of breasts, heart, chest and pelvis. The patient is asked by the nurse to undress, leaving on only her pants, and is requested to lie on a couch and given a cover blanket.

Afterwards the weight and blood pressure are recorded and the urine tested for albumen and sugar. Blood is taken by the nurse for haemoglobin—5 ml in a sequestrene bottle; grouping and WR—10 ml clotted and 5 ml in a sequestrene bottle; rubella antibodies—5 ml clotted blood (if not previously recorded).

The appropriate booking for home, GP unit or hospital confinement is arranged and the patient is given an exemption certificate for free dental care and free prescriptions. Relaxation, baby- and parent-craft classes can be arranged, advice and education given about breast or bottle feeding and counselling about smoking, drinking and diet is given by the midwife or practice nurse. Useful booklets on pregnancy and the confinement should be available. The patient then returns for further antenatal visits at monthly intervals until 28 weeks pregnant. At these visits the weight and blood pressure are recorded and the urine tested for albumen and sugar by the midwife or practice nurse and the patient examined by the doctor and/or midwife. From the 28th week of pregnancy the patient is seen every two weeks, and from 36 weeks to term she is seen weekly.

Haemoglobin estimation is repeated by the midwife or practice nurse at about 30 and 36 weeks of pregnancy and blood taken for Rhesus incompatability at 32 weeks in those patients where it is indicated.

Postnatal clinics

The patient attends for her full postnatal examination about six weeks after confinement. In most practices antenatal and postnatal patients are seen at the same clinic. At this visit baby management problems and contraception are discussed by the doctor, midwife and practice nurse. The routine of weight, BP and urine testing are followed and the haemoglobin checked. If the patient was rubella susceptible this vaccine can now be given by the practice nurse. The patient is then prepared for examination. A routine cervical smear is taken at this time. A trolley or tray with vaginal speculae, Ayres spatula for cervical smear, container with industrial methylated spirit, disposable gloves and lubricant jelly should be set ready with the appropriate forms completed by the midwife or practice nurse. The doctor should also complete the maternity claim form FP24 for the services performed during the pregnancy.

The subject of contraception should also be discussed. The patient can be started on oral contraceptives immediately or, if breast feeding, given the progestogen-only pill (e.g. Noriday—see Chapter 10). Advice on other methods of contraception can be given, and an IUCD or cap can be fitted if this is appropriate. Form FP1001 should be signed by the patient obtaining contraceptive advice and services. After the postnatal examination the nurse may encourage the patient to continue postnatal exercises to regain muscle tone.

(a) Lie on couch, lift both legs straight up, slowly lower to the couch, repeat ten times twice daily.
(b) During micturation, stop midstream for a short while, then complete the stream.
(c) Tighten the buttock and perineal muscles when standing (this can be performed often, even at a sink doing household chores).

Opportunity should not be lost for giving health education about smoking and obesity, and advice about the baby's future immunisations.

It should be emphasised that in the antenatal and postnatal clinics the practice nurse's role is to support and complement the work of the doctor, midwife and health visitor by being available to help if a clinic becomes very busy or if the midwife is unavailable. At the postnatal examination the practice nurse with her expertise in family planning will be involved in counselling and advice for future baby injections.

Some practices take their routine cervical smears at specific clinics organised once or twice a month. It is more likely that this type of preventive care may be incorporated into a well woman clinic.

Breast self-examination can be taught at this time or at any other appropriate opportunity.

Breast examination

Routine examination of the breasts can be included when a female patient visits the surgery for any other purpose, such as for contraception or a routine cervical smear. The practice nurse is of particular value as she can examine the patient's breasts and then spend time teaching each patient the routine of self-examination.

It is important to explain to the patient the importance of regular self-examination of the breasts, reassuring her that the vast majority of irregularities or lumps in the breast are non-malignant, but that if she detects anything abnormal she should not hesitate to seek advice. When performing regular self-examination the patient gets to know the normal feel of her breast tissue and then if any abnormality is felt it can be detected at an early stage. Women should be encouraged to examine their breasts monthly immediately after their menstrual period, when the breasts are usually at their softest and least hormonally active. If the patient is no longer having menstrual periods she should be advised to select the same day each month so the examination is not forgotten.

There are two stages in examining the breast tissue.

1   Looking at the breasts.
2   Feeling the breast tissue.

1   *Looking at the breasts*

The patient is asked to undress to the waist and to let her arms hang loosely to the side, then to raise her arms above her head. The nurse explains the reasons to the patient for doing this.

(a)   To notice any changes in the size of either breast.
(b)   To note any changes, bleeding or discharge from either nipple.
(c)   To note any unusual dimple or puckering on the breast or nipple.
(d)   To look for any veins standing out more than is usual in the breasts.

These observations can be performed in front of a mirror when a patient is examining herself at home.

2   *Feeling the breast tissue*

Lay the patient on a couch or bed with one pillow under her head, lift the right arm above the head and examine the right breast, then the left arm above the head to examine the left breast. When the patient examines herself at home the left hand examines the right breast and vice versa.

When feeling the breast tissue the fingers are kept together and the flat part of the fingers only are used for feeling each quadrant. Each breast can be divided into four quadrants. Starting with the upper inner quadrant guide the flat part of fingers from outside towards the nipple. In the same way take each of the other quadrants in turn until all of each breast has been felt. The nipple should then be squeezed gently to check for any discharge or bleeding. Finally the axillae should be examined, still using the flat part of the fingers, working down towards the breast to check for any irregularities in the lymph glands. A number of helpful patient booklets have been published by the Health Education Council and other organisations. Having these available to give to the patient will reinforce your advice.

Child development clinic

For many years the prime responsibility for routine examination of children has been undertaken by the local authority in their child development and school clinics. There has been an increasing demand for these activities to be undertaken by the general practitioner and many doctors run developmental assessment or 'well baby' clinics, sometimes in conjunction with the immunisation sessions.

The practice nurse may be involved in these clinics when either giving the immunisations or in assisting the health visitor in the counselling of young mothers. The child will be sent for at certain specified times during its early childhood for review of its development, and to give the mother an opportunity to discuss any problems which she may have and which she felt inappropriate to discuss in a routine appointment during normal surgery consultation hours.

There is debate as to the value of examining children frequently— as with most situations, the families who need the support and supervision are the ones least likely to present themselves. In circumstances where the child is not brought to the surgery for these assessments the health visitor will visit the child at home. An example is shown of a developmental assessment record such as might be used in such a clinic (Appendix III).

Significant undiscovered abnormalities are infrequently found during the examination, but there is no doubt that meeting their mothers and children in this way increases the relationship between doctor/nurse and patient. The practice will need to be organised to accommodate this extra work, but some appointments will be saved as mothers will not then need to come to surgery to discuss a problem which is not urgent.

The Royal College of General Practitioners identifies twenty areas where intervention may make a dramatic difference to the consequences of a child's development—it is worth doctor and nurse bearing these in mind when seeing children at any time.

The areas are:

1   Contraception (adult)
2   Encouraging breast feeding
3   Discouraging smoking (adult)
4   Antenatal care
5   Chemical screening (e.g. phenylketonuria)
6   Congenital dislocation of the hip
7   Maldescent of the testes (boys)
8   Polio immunisation
9   Tetanus immunisation
10 Diphtheria immunisation
11 Pertussis immunisation
12 Measles immunisation
13 Hearing
14 Squint
15 Visual acuity
16 Colour vision

17   Rubella (girls)
18   Scoliosis
19   Discouraging smoking (child)
20   Contraception (child)

The height and weight are also recorded on a percentile chart which shows where these measurements are in relation to normal children of the same age and sex. Using a percentile chart can demonstrate readily when a child's development is falling off in relation to his or her peers or to their previous records.

Developmental assessment charts and percentile charts are shown in Appendix III and IV.

Child abuse

The nurse must always be alert to the possibility of non accidental injury in a child. As she may see the child more frequently than other members of the primary health care team she must bear this in mind and note any abnormal or frequent injuries; particularly those with specific significance such as small circular burns (cigarettes), bruises suggestive of fingertip grasp (upper arms) or from blows—ears and lips. The relationship between the child and the mother should also be noted.

The recent rise in cases of recognised and reported child sexual abuse has highlighted an area in which doctor and nurse will have to be particularly vigilant. This can occur at any age or social class and in either sex but is more likely in girls between the ages of eight and 16 years. Any suggestion of sexual abuse from physical findings or, more usually, verbal comments, should be taken seriously. It is obviously important to deal with these matters confidentially and sensitively because producing definite evidence is often extremely difficult.

Because of her close relationship with the family the practice nurse will often be familiar with the background and problems of her families and be already aware of those at risk from various factors such as poverty, stress or alcoholism.

However, it should be borne in mind that the incidence of abuse in children covers all social classes and if the nurse has the slightest suspicion she should discuss it with the doctor or health visitor and certainly not dismiss the possibility out of hand.

Family planning clinics

Family planning clinics are discussed in Chapter 10.

GROUP (2) CLINICS

Diabetic clinic

Patients attending diabetic clinics in general practice can be divided into two categories:

1 Those who are requiring regular insulin—usually children or younger adults.
2 Mature patients controlled on diet alone or controlled on diet and oral hypoglycaemic agents.

1 *Children and adults dependent on insulin and diet*

Patients have often been hospitalised for preliminary adjustment of their diet and insulin, and are also taught self-administration of injections and urine testing. After discharge from the hospital these patients need support and help from their GP and the practice nurse. The names of diabetic patients should be entered in a specific register or on the practice computer system so that diabetic patients can be recalled (Chapter 2). It is important that all diabetic patients in the practice can be readily identified if effective supervision of their management is to occur. Each member of the practice team must understand their role in this supervision.

The patients may then be reviewed as discussed below, although if they are regularly attending hospital their practice surveillance may be modified.

If the diabetic patient is a child or young person, parent involvement is very important. The practice nurse should encourage the parent or guardian to attend at each visit, so that any problems, especially dietary, can be discussed. A check should be made on the dose of insulin, the sites used for injection and whether the patient is managing to cope well with the self-administration of injections. It is helpful for the parents of children to be taught the routine of administration of the insulin so they can aid the child in the early stages of the illness. Advice about hypoglycaemia attacks will be found in Chapter 8.

2   Mature patients controlled on diet or on diet and oral hypoglycaemic agents: Non-insulin dependent diabetes

Patients who develop diabetes in later life are often anxious about the consequences of the disease. They have usually presented themselves to the doctor with symptoms of thirst, general malaise or tiredness. Sometimes there is a superadded infection and often the patients are obese. Sometimes glycosuria is an unexpected finding on routine urine testing. When diabetes is diagnosed these patients can often be regulated and controlled on diet alone or diet and oral hypoglycaemic agents such as tolbutamide or glibenclamide. Rarely do these mature onset diabetics need insulin but they can still develop the complications of the disease.

At the initial consultation, after detection of glycosuria by testing the urine:

The nurse's role

1   General discussion and explanation about diabetes.
2   Weight, height, blood pressure measurement.
3   Teach the patient urine testing—using diastix or clinistix.
4   Give a record book to the patient for urine tests and start a cooperation card (see Appendix V).
5   Take blood for measurement of glucose, creatinine and glycosylated haemoglobin or fructisamine.
6   Teach the patient how to manage their diet (an example is given in Appendix VI).
7   Give the information to the doctor.

The doctor's role

1   To check that the patient understands instruction and advice already received.
2   Clinical examination, including eyes and feet.
3   Start any treatment and diet.
4   Arrange next appointment.

A diabetic record book such as provided to the patient by the nurse is seen in Appendix V.

Patients should be encouraged initially to test their urine twice daily, the first time before breakfast, the second before retiring to bed. It is beneficial for patients to keep urine testing equipment on a tray used only for this purpose and the nurse should explain the purpose and the dosage of tablets, if these are required, and confirm that the patient understands the instructions. Regular home monitoring of blood sugar should be taught.

A regular visit to the chiropodist for foot care is advised, as diabetics often experience poor circulation of the extremities. In circumstances when the patient does not visit the chiropodist the practice nurse will check the feet for any abnormalities at the routine visit.

Regular eye and teeth check-ups are recommended.

The practice nurse should then see the patient at weekly intervals until she is confident that the patient is well regulated and managing the urine and blood testing. He or she can then be seen at less frequent intervals, according to the practice routine.

When attending for an annual review the patient should be warned that the pupils will be dilated so that they will be unable to drive for several hours. It is usually best if a friend or relative accompanies them in these circumstances.

The security to the patients of knowing that they can always come and discuss their management problems with the nurse is invaluable.

Established diabetics and follow up clinics

1   Check the patient is on the recall diabetic register or computer.
2   Decide how frequently the patient is to be seen, i.e. 3–6 monthly.

For the routine clinic

Secretary
1   Make appointments.
2   Prepare notes and complete routine prescriptions requests.

Practice Nurse
1   Discuss any worries.
2   Discuss diet.
3   Weight.
4   Test urine for glucose, ketones, protein.
5   Take blood sugar and glycosylated Hb or fructosamine.
6   Record information on co-operation card.

Doctor
1   Review treatment and results.
2   Discuss any problems or symptoms.
3   Check any change in eyes or feet.
4   Appropriate examination.
5   Arrange next appointment.

For the annual review

Secretary
1 Send appointment letter.
2 Prepare notes.

Practice Nurse
1 As for routine clinic review.
2 Visual acuity including using pinhole card.
3 Instill tropicamide to both eyes (to dilate the pupils).
4 Blood pressure.
5 Examine feet—general, footwear, pulses.
6 Bloods—creatinine, glycosylated Hb, blood sugar fructosamine.
7 Check diet and education.
8 Smoking and drinking advice.
9 Record on co-operation cards.

Doctor
1 As for Routine Clinic review.
2 Examine the dilated eyes.
3 Discuss any problems and make further appointment.

Some dietary guidelines for diabetic patients can be found in Appendix VI but each patient must be advised individually.

This is only a suggested supervision regimen for diabetic patients. Some practices will wish to supervise their diabetic patients completely and others will wish to share this responsibility with the hospital specialist. Either method does not matter as long as the patient gets the best possible care and does not fall through the net and miss having early diabetic complications identified at a time when action is possible to halt or reduce the problem. This is especially true for diabetic retinopathy which may be severe before the patient has any symptoms.

Hypertension clinics

Hypertensive patients are referred from the GP. When dealing with these patients the GP and practice nurse must fully discuss the guidelines and routine procedures to be followed and it is best if the practice has a management plan for this.

A suggested protocol is as follows:

Requirements for running a hypertensive clinic in general practice

The practice nurse can effectively participate in the initial assessment and follow up care of hypertensive patients. She needs to be motivated and interested in preventive medicine, have space available and agreement from all the partners.

Screening

A register can be compiled of all known hypertensive patients, similar to the diabetic register. Patients may be identified when they present symptomatically or opportunistically if the practice has a policy of recording the blood pressure of all patients between the ages of 40–65 at a surgery visit if this has not been done. They may also be identified from a well man or well woman clinic.

Patients found to have raised blood pressure

Pre-treatment checks
1   Take three B/P readings and calculate mean reading.
2   Check history.
3   Check and advise on risk factors.

If the average diastolic reading is less than 100 mm
Advice is given about any risk factors, i.e. smoking/weight/alcohol/salt intake and a further appointment to see the nurse in six months for blood pressure check is made.

If diastolic reading is more than 100 mm
Practice nurse
   (a)   The nurse records in the patients notes
      (i)   Weight
      (ii)   Smoking
      (iii)   Alcohol
      (iv)   Urinalysis
      (v)   Renal function tests and creatinine
      (vi)   Serum lipids
      (vii)   ECG result

A specific record card or rubber stamp in the notes if helpful.

   (b)   Advice is given on diet, salt intake, stress, exercise, smoking and alcohol.

(c)   The patient then makes an appointment to see the general practitioner two weeks later.

Doctor
(a)   The results of the investigations are discussed and assessed.
(b)   Medical examination especially of cardiovascular system and retina.
(c)   Decides if treatment is needed or risk factors to be modified.
(d)   Decides target weight and blood pressure.
(e)   Discuss with the practice nurse the follow-up arrangements.
(f)   Further appointment made with nurse or doctor.

If blood pressure is under control
The practice nurse can review six monthly for blood pressure, weight and urinalysis.

If blood pressure is raised
General practitioner initiates drug treatment and patient is reviewed in one month.

Annual reviews

If blood pressure under control:
1   Take two BP readings and calculate mean pressure.
2   Check weight.
3   Check compliance.
4   Check pulse rate (if beta blocker is used).
5   Check any side effects from drugs i.e. nausea, diarrhoea, giddiness, lassitude, faintness, impotence, cold extremities.
6   Check risk factor.
7   Consult doctor if BP not at target level.
8   Give appointment for next visit.

A possible flow chart for this type of practice management plan is shown in Appendix VII. The nurse must be aware of the blood pressure levels at which she is expected to refer the patient back to the doctor and the levels at which she can make her own decisons on treatment.

The nurse may be given some discretion for modifying treatment slightly, (e.g. adding another diuretic tablet) but this is obviously an individual decision. Her main function is to monitor the levels in a less stressful environment and to reduce the frequency with which the patient needs to see the doctor. These meetings with the nurse give the patient an opportunity to ventilate any further anxieties which he or she may have.

Asthma clinic

In general practice, care of the asthmatic patient can be shared with the doctor by an appropriately trained nurse. Courses are now available to practice nurses run by the Asthma Training Centre. These courses prepare and teach nurses to run asthma clinics in general practice and are an exciting extension of the practice nurse role.

Necessary requirements for a nurse to run an asthma clinic are:

1 Specially trained nurse who is enthusiastic.
2 General practitioners who are keen to support her.
3 Effective record systems i.e. computer or card index, with a register of asthma patients.
4 Plan for diagnosis and treatment.
5 Time and space.
6 Follow-up protocol.

Starting an asthma clinic

1 Compile a register of all asthma patients in the practice. This can be done by computer, opportunistic screening, repeat prescriptions or by checking all the notes.
2 The doctor and practice nurse will decide which patients will benefit from attending the clinic.

Suggested protocol for running an asthma clinic
1 The nurse must gain patient confidence, so enough time must be allocated to explain about the clinic and its objectives.
2 Prepare a record card—(suggested format may be obtained from The Asthma Society) or a record card can be prepared by the practice nurse.
3 Measure peak flow.
4 Measure height and weight of patient.
5 Check
   (a) History
   (b) Present symptoms
   (c) Asthma state
   (d) Asthma treatment
   (e) Other medical conditions, treatment and investigations
6 Discuss with the general practitioner the findings and treatment.

7 Give patient
   (a) Treatment and treatment card record
   (b) Instruction booklet
   (c) Peak flow and chart (if home monitoring)
   (d) Next appointment

Follow-up clinic

1 After the initial visit the patient should be seen after one week to check the state of patient and technique of treatment.
2 The follow-up patient can be seen three monthly or well-controlled mild asthmatics can be seen annually.
3 All patients must be encouraged to contact the practice if there are persistent symptoms or if the peak flow reading drops significantly.

At the follow-up clinic
Check
   (a) Symptoms
   (b) Home monitoring results
   (c) Inhalation technique
   (d) Discuss treatment and give new record card
   (e) Next appointment

The practice nurse can be involved in asthma care in general practice in many different forms from:

Minimum involvement—Setting up register:
         to   Record peak flow and demonstrate inhaler technique

Maximum involvement—Assessment and follow up:
                          Formulate treatment plan
                          Prepare prescriptions
                          Advice over the telephone
                          See patients in an emergency with the doctor

GROUP (3) CLINICS

Obesity clinics

Overweight patients will often lose weight when encouraged to do so by an enthusiastic practice nurse. The nurse may motivate the patient by telling him or her of the health risks of obesity. Encouragement about appearance and clothes will often help the female patients to feel more confident. The patients may refer themselves to the nurse for help, or alternatively be told by the GP that their health is at risk if they do not lose weight.

At the initial consultation the practice nurse finds out the patient's occupation, social and family background. The patient is weighed, measured and advised on the amount of weight loss at which to aim. One record card is given to the patient and one retained in the treatment room for reference. The patient is advised to return for weighing at weekly intervals for the first two months. After a steady loss is recorded the patient can then return monthly until the target weight is achieved. Thereafter the patient should return at six monthly intervals for encouragement and to try and prevent a slow return to the previous weight level.

A suitable diet is worked out for each patient. There are many reducing diets, some more exotic than others. It is important that the type of diet chosen for the patient can be incorporated into a family menu at little extra expense, and a full time working patient should have a diet which provides enough calories for his or her energy expenditure. For these reasons a very successful diet is based on 1000 calories per day. Divide the calories into three sections, three hundred for breakfast, three hundred for lunch and three hundred for the evening meal, leaving one hundred calories for fluid intake during the day. Patients using this form of diet should be encouraged to calorie count for each day, making sure that a balanced diet is taken. Calorie diet sheets can be obtained from most Area Health Authorities, health education offices, or the dietician at a local hospital. Some drug firms also produce very good diet sheets (see Appendix VIII). In the past few years various specialised extremely low calorie diets such as the Cambridge Diet have been introduced. These diets do have a part to play in refractory obesity but can produce severe physiological changes and need to be supervised carefully. Patients who only need to lose twenty pounds or less certainly should not be encouraged to use this type of diet.

For less obese patients, simple control of the carbohydrates taken in the form of chips, sweets, puddings or sugar is often sufficient to cause weight reduction. Alcohol is also a contributing cause to obesity, particularly in men, and reduction or abolition of any daily intake will be sufficient in itself to bring the weight down to a reasonable level.

It is now recognised that obese patients are not necessarily overeating but that their metabolism and family history will play a significant part in their weight gain. They can still lose weight if given enough encouragement but it will be difficult for them.

Stopping smoking

There is increasing pressure upon smokers to stop and this may result in patients either being referred by the GP or seeking help from the nurse directly. In either instance the practice nurse must be prepared to spend time explaining the dangers to health and the social aspects of smoking and how she can assist the patient to stop smoking.

The dangers to health

1 Bronchitis.
2 Emphysema.
3 Heart disease and hypertension.
4 Peripheral vascular disease.
5 Cancer of lung, throat, tongue and mouth.
6 Peptic and duodenal ulceration.
7 Pregnant women more likely to have smaller, unhealthy babies.
8 Children growing up in an environment where the parents smoke more likely to have respiratory infections.

Often patients have symptoms of some of these conditions before they ask for help but it must be impressed on the patient that it is never too late to give up smoking and it can be a very important way of improving health.

Social aspects of smoking

1 Constant smell of smoke on clothes, body, breath and hair.
2 Cost.
3 Very antisocial habit.
4 Children follow the example of their parents and peers.

Routine for breaking the habit of smoking

1 Choose a date in the next few days, avoiding a day likely to be stressful.
2 Make a definite decision on date and time to stop.
3 Tell people in close contact of the decision to stop smoking and try to persuade someone else to give up smoking at the same time.
4 The evening before the 'big' day smoke the last cigarette and then throw the remaining cigarettes away.

Helpful hints for the new non-smoker

1 Avoid temptation—put ashtrays, matches and cigarettes out of sight.
2 Keep away from smokers.
3 Change habits, avoid breaks when usually a cigarette is smoked.
4 Keep supply of chewing gum, apple or carrot to nibble if necessary.
5 Put aside the money which is saved each day.
6 Think of all the good reasons for giving up smoking.
7 Never be tempted to have just one cigarette.
8 If you succumb and find you have lit a cigarette, immediately put it out, but this is the cigarette which must be lit first next time you feel like having one.

Nicotine chewing gum (nicorette) may be a useful support during the early stages of withdrawal and can be prescribed as a private prescription. It costs about the same for each packet as 20 cigarettes and should be used when the desire to smoke is intense. Full instructions are given with each packet.

Helpful leaflets and literature can be obtained from the Health Education Council.

Well women/men clinics

Patients are now more conscious of health, health education and preventive care and practices may now be taking advantage of this.

The running of preventive care activities within the practice requires the resources of the whole team. The doctors will need to decide on priority groups (e.g. mean aged 40–60) and the receptionists, practice nurses and, possibly, health visitors will be involved in making these clinics successful.

Patients may know that a well woman/man clinic is organised and ask if they may attend. Care must be taken to see that those traditionally seeking this type of supervision (middle aged social class I and II women) are not the only ones encouraged to attend.

Practice recall systems can identify groups at risk or specific age/sex groups and a policy instituted of writing to those in the group inviting them to attend a clinic. Non-responders should be followed up but not exhaustively as the right to refuse this type of intervention should be respected.

Suggested format for well women clinic

1 Smear

2   Breast check and teaching self examination
3   Weight and diet
4   Tetanus and polio state
5   Exercise
6   Smoking
7   Alcohol
8   Blood pressure

Suggested format for well men Clinic

1   Blood pressure
2   Weight and diet
3   Smoking
4   Alcohol
5   Exercise
6   Tetanus and polio state

Advice on further follow-up can be taken depending on the results of these investigations.

FURTHER READING

Pearson R. *Asthma Care in General Practice.* Asthma Society Training Centre, Stratford on Avon.

Pyne Reginald H. (1981) *Professional Discipline in Nursing.* Blackwell Scientific Publications, Oxford.

RCGP (1982) *Healthier Children Thinking Prevention.* Occasional Paper 22.

The Royal College of Nursing of the United Kingdom (1979) *The Extended Clinical Role of the Nurse.*

The Royal College of Nursing of the United Kingdom (1980) *Drug Administration—A Nursing Responsibility.*

The Royal College of Nursing of the United Kingdom (1980) *Guidelines on Confidentiality in Nursing.*

The Royal College of Nursing of the United Kingdom publications.

(a)   *RCN advice to Practice/Treatment Room Nurses* (April 1980)
(b)   *Guidelines on Immunisation and Vaccination*
(c)   *The GP Employed Practice Nurse.*

Skeet Muriel (1981) *Emergency Procedures and First Aid for Nurses.* Blackwell Scientific Publications, Oxford.

The Clinic Handbook for Family Planning Nurses. Published by: The Family Planning Association, 27/35 Mortimer Street, London.

Chapter 12

Prescribing and Management Advice

The practice nurse is not allowed by law to sign prescriptions, but there are many occasions on which she will be asked advice by patients about their prescriptions, and some occasions where she will have assessed a patient and be able, with the doctor, to decide the most appropriate treatment.

There are some parts of the world where paramedical personnel do have a limited prescribing function (e.g. the nurse practitioner in the USA). Some discussion has taken place in the UK about giving nurses with family planning training limited prescribing powers in this field, but progress is likely to be slow as the medical profession is reluctant to admit that anyone other than a doctor could prescribe for a patient.

Responsibilities

1 To ensure that the correct prescription is given to the correct patient, or patient's representative, where appropriate.
2 To be able to answer knowledgeably, and give simple advice to patients who may make enquiries about their medication.
3 To ensure that no abuse of drugs occurs within her range of responsibility and that prescription pads in the treatment room are not accessible to patients.
4 To be familiar with repeat prescribing systems.
5 To be familiar with the availability of drug information and to have appropriate reference books to hand.

A few of these responsibilities will now be looked at in more detail.

Access to drugs

The regulations concerning the Misuse of Drugs Act are discussed later in the chapter. The nurse must carry the key to the dangerous drugs cupboard and be responsible for checking out any drugs issued.

In addition, prescriptions and prescription pads can be stolen by those passing through if left lying around in the treatment room.

Patients who are having a course of injections (e.g. cyatamen or depixol) must be given a prescription from the doctor for the injection and obtain these from the chemist before returning to the nurse to commence or continue the course. The nurse may choose to keep these injections in the treatment room during the course, and if they are to be continued, she may obtain the prescription in advance from the doctor before supplies are exhausted.

Repeat prescribing system

Many practices have some sort of system whereby patients requiring a repeat medication for a chronic ailment can obtain it without necessarily seeing the doctor. Whatever the method used the basic principles are the same:

1 The patient and the doctor should already have agreed which drugs can be on repeat prescription.
2 A card should be issued stating the drug, dose, strength and quantity to be dispensed and date issued.
3 All repeat prescription requests should be entered in the patient's record. The implication of this is that there has to be a stop date written on the repeat prescription card and also in the notes and that the staff have to take action when that stop date is reached. The doctor's attention should be drawn to the fact and it is then his or her decision whether to extend the repeat prescription time to a new stop date, or see the patient before another prescription is issued.

Although the administration of this system is essentially a secretarial one the nurse should be familiar with it as queries and questions will often come to her. Patients may well ask for a repeat prescription when visiting the practice nurse.

Drugs available from the chemist

The number of effective drugs available over the chemist's counter changes periodically and more have become available since the introduction of the restricted prescribing list by the DHSS which prohibited many commonly prescribed medications from being prescribed on an FP10. The introduction of the restricted list has made little practical difference to the doctor as it was principally aimed at the wide variety of proprietary brand medicines available for minor illness. These brands can often be purchased by the patient and to some extent has rationalised what was essentially a rather random process of prescribing.

The nurse should have a good relationship with her local chemist or chemists and know what commonly used preparations such as antacids, antihistamines and cough linctuses are available and approximately how much they will cost. She can then advise patients who ask her opinion about self-medication and also have someone she can turn to for advice on these matters. As cost is a major factor in the medication she should also know those patients on low-income supplements and other social security benefits and ensure that they are aware that they may qualify for free prescriptions. In this case it will be to the patient's financial advantage to have a prescription issued, even for something simple like aspirin, rather than purchase it.

Reference books

The two main books which should always be available in the treatment room are the *British National Formulary* (BNF) and the *Monthly Index of Medical Specialities* (MIMS). The *British National Formulary* is a small book packed with information about the commonly used drugs, their indications and contraindications and a guide to the relative cost of them. It is issued free to all general practitioners by the DHSS via the Family Practitioner Committee. The *Monthly Index of Medical Specialities* is a comprehensive list of all the proprietary preparations available on prescription. There is a brief outline of indications and contraindications, plus detailed information, in prescribing and cost. It is issued independently and financed by the drug advertising which it includes. There is no indication of which drugs or preparations are more appropriate than another for a specific condition, and therefore is only of use as a reference book to check on a known preparation. It is published and distributed free to all general practitioners monthly, on the basis that proprietary preparations are changing all the time. Previous publications are supposed to be destroyed when a new one arrives.

Controlled drugs

From time to time the practice nurse may have to handle controlled drugs and many practices will keep their stock of drugs in the treatment room. Because of this it is important for the nurse to be aware of the regulations concerning this group of drugs. They are outlined in the Misuse of Drugs Regulations (1973) and the principle legal requirements are that:

1   The prescription must be signed in full (not initialled) and dated by the prescriber.
2   It must have the prescriber's address on it.
3   The prescriber must write the prescription in his or her own handwriting and in an indelible ink.
4   It must contain the name and address of the patient.
5   The quantity and dose of the drug must be written in both words and numbers.

The Misuse of Drugs Act (1971)

The Misuse of Drugs Act (1971) was the successor to the original Dangerous Drug Act and was intended to provide more flexible and comprehensive control over the misuse of drugs of all kinds. The drugs concerned are divided into three categories according to the harmfulness of the drug when it is misused:
Class A cocaine, diamorphine (heroin), dipipanone, methadone, morphine and pethidine.
Class B oral amphetamines, cannabis, codeine and pholcodeine.
Class C certain drugs related to the amphetamines.

In addition, the regulations require a medical practitioner to notify the Chief Medical Officer, Drugs Branch, Queen Anne's Gate, London, of any person he or she considers to be addicted to a number of substances which include cocaine, diamorphine and pethidine. There are other regulations concerning the notification of addicts which do not need to concern the practice nurse but further details are given in the *British National Formulary* if she is interested. Prescriptions for registered drug addicts under treatment have to be written on a yellow FP10.

Further regulations which do concern her are those about the storage and recording of drugs. Controlled drugs must always be kept in a locked cupboard and a register of drugs kept on the premises. This register will note any new stock and when it was obtained, and will record the dispensing of this stock to patients or to individual doctors for their emergency bag.

Nurses should be particularly careful that prescription pads, in the treatment room for the convenience of the doctors, are not left lying around where they may be stolen by patients. Obviously, care should be taken with any other drugs which may be kept in the treatment room but which do not fall into the categories described in the Misuse of Drugs Regulation.

GENERAL PRINCIPLES OF TAKING DRUGS

The practice nurse will frequently be asked for advice by the patient about drugs which he or she is taking. These drugs may be prescribed by the doctor or purchased over the chemist's counter. There are a number of principles with which the nurse should be familiar if she is to be able to offer meaningful advice to these patients.

1 The instructions for prescribed drugs should be clearly indicated on the prescription and on the container in which they are dispensed. The nurse should check to see that the patient fully understands these when they are dispensed in connection with a condition which she is involved in treating.
2 Many drugs interact with alcohol and it is a good principle to advise patients to avoid it while on treatment.
3 Some drugs need to be taken with food or they irritate the bowel and other drugs need to be taken on an empty stomach to facilitate absorption. If there is any doubt about the drug in relationship to food the nurse should ask the doctor or check the BNF.
4 Some drugs such as anticoagulants and steroids need careful monitoring and an awareness by the patient of the importance of this. All patients taking these groups of drugs should be issued with the appropriate instruction booklet. Many other foodstuffs and drugs interact with these groups so great care must be taken in advising these patients accordingly.
5 If a drug (for example penicillin) has to be taken four times a day it is important that the dosage is spread through the 24 hours evenly as far as possible. The value of an antibiotic is considerably reduced if four doses are crammed into 12 hours of each day as might well happen in the case of a child. Parents should be told to wake the child if necessary for the last dose of the day when they go to bed, not to give the last dose when the child goes to bed. For this reason antibiotics which only have to be given twice or three times a day may be preferred and improve patients compliance.

There follows a description of some of the more common conditions with the drugs and advice which might be given. The list is neither comprehensive nor exclusive and for more detailed information the reader is referred to books which are entirely about prescribing.

COMMON CONDITIONS WITH THEIR DRUG TREATMENT

Acne

The spotty skin which comes with adolescence is often a great source of anxiety and embarrassment to the teenager. Because of this embarrassment they often will not seek advice but spend a great deal of money on proprietary over-the-counter preparations.

Preparations used in treating acne aim at reducing the grease in the skin and reducing the number of blocked sebaceous ducts (blackheads). Desquamatory agents include Quinoderm, Dome-acne cleanser and Retin A. They can all make the skin rather sore and treatment should be stopped for a few days if this occurs.

Application of one preparation containing multiple constituents such as Neomedrone acne lotion is probably best avoided as they contain sensitising agents such as neomycin and also a steroid.

In severe acne with persistent pustules and spots on the face and shoulders the doctor may prescribe oxytetracycline or erythromycin 250 mg tablets in a dose of up to four tablets daily. Although it is an antibiotic the drug is not used only for this purpose, but is thought to have a specific action on the cells in the lower layers of the skin to make them less prone to produce the pustule formation. It is certainly effective but needs to be taken for several months at least.

Precautions

The tetracycline group of drugs is best absorbed if taken on an empty stomach half an hour before meals. For the same reason milk drinks inhibit absorption. This group also produce photosensitivity in some people and patients should be warned that their skin may become unduly sensitive on prolonged exposure to sunshine. This last effect should be borne in mind as the cheapest form of treatment for acne is exposure to the ultraviolet light of the sun and encouragement to expose the skin at every opportunity should be given. However, teenagers already ashamed of their appearance may not always heed this advice.

General advice

Young patients with severe acne often need a lot of support and counselling. They should be encouraged to lead a normal social life, and not to use make-up to cover their blemishes as this will block sebaceous ducts even more and aggravate the situation.

A diet high in carbohydrates and fats is also thought to aggravate the condition. Of course many teenagers like fried foods, chips, cakes and chocolate which should be avoided. General advice about diet and the value of non greasy foods and fresh fruit should be emphasised as part of a general pattern of health education in the practice.

Allergies

There are many causes of allergies such as reactions to insect bites, pollen, drugs or foodstuffs, but the symptoms are often similar. Skin irritation, rashes (particularly on the extremities) and catarrhal reactions are among the symptoms of these unfortunate patients.

While part of the treatment should be directed towards seeking the cause of the allergy, a number of drugs will reduce the symptoms.

Antihistamines

Antihistamines are a large group of drugs which include chlorpheniramine (Piriton) and promethazine (Phenergan). Some of them may be purchased over the counter at the pharmacy. The dose of chlorpheniramine syrup for children is up to 5 ml three times a day, according to age; promethazine is more sedative and tends to be given in 5 to 10 ml dosages, at night, for decongestion of the nasal airways. The comparable adult dose is 5 mg three times a day for chlorpheniramine and 10–25 mg of promethazine at night.

Precautions

All antihistamines tend to produce drowsiness and a dry mouth so those patients driving cars or working with machinery should be warned about this. Patients tend to be very individual in their reactions to antihistamines; since there are many varieties available it is worth trying different ones if side-effects are unacceptable. MIMS will give a comprehensive list of those available. Some preparations are slow release ones which only need to be taken once a day and often have a lower incidence of side effects.

Depot steroid preparations

Some doctors prescribe a depot steroid at the start of the hay fever season for patients. This is a long acting steroid which will not provoke an anaphylactic reaction, so the precautions for densensitising injections do not apply. The nurse should clarify the situation with the doctor if she is unsure.

Angina

The characteristic pain of angina is caused by increased workload upon the heart muscle when the coronary circulation is not adequate to respond to the demand. The pain tends to be retrosternal and may radiate into the neck and shoulders, and may also go down the left arm. It is precipitated by effort and will settle quickly when this is stopped. Any pain which does not settle very quickly when the patient rests must be viewed with caution since angina is only a symptom of coronary insufficiency and a complete myocardial infarction may occur. Conversely pain which is worse at rest is unlikely to be angina.

Glyceryl trinitrate

It has been in use for many years for angina and is still popular today. It acts by temporarily improving the blood supply to the myocardium. This results in better oxygenation of the heart muscle and the pain goes. Glyceryl trinitrate (trinitrin) has to be absorbed under the tongue as it is inactivated by the gastric juices. It has a short duration of action (only five or ten minutes) so it is a very safe drug to take in repeated doses. Patients should be encouraged to carry their tablets everywhere and to use them as frequently as they need to do so. They should also use them prophylactically to prevent an attack coming on (e.g. when climbing stairs).

There are some long-acting trinitrin preparations now available which may reduce the need for frequent use of glyceryl trinitrate tablets. The only side-effect which some patients have is that the drug will dilate the cerebral vessels as well as the coronary ones and produce an intense headache. Occasionally patients will have to stop using trinitrin because of this but the headaches do recede quickly as the action of the drug is short.

Patches impregnated with a drug stuck to the skin, so that transdermal absorption reduces the need for oral medication, have been introduced but their value at present is not proven.

Beta blockers

Dramatic changes in the management of a number of conditions related to the circulation have occurred in the last ten or fifteen years as a result of the introduction of the beta blocker group of drugs. The commonly used ones are propranolol (Inderal), atenolol (Tenormin) and oxprenolol (Transicor). They act by blocking nerve transmission at the myoneural junction to the various receptors there. In angina, they work by reducing the muscle demand and hence the oxygen requirement which means that the pain will not come on so readily.

If patients are bordering on heart failure or have asthma they are contraindicated but further details of action and side-effects is beyond the scope of this book.

Anticoagulants

Patients will be discharged from hospital on anticoagulants following deep vein thrombosis, cardiac surgery, myocardial infarction and other conditions where clotting of the blood presents problems. The two main drugs used are warfarin or phenindione (Dindevan) and the dose must be tailored to the individual patient. Their action is complex; many other drugs and some foods will potentiate or reduce this, making patients more or less anticoagulated. A table of drug interactions will be found in the BNF.

Precautions

Patients should be warned against taking aspirin, which might cause gastrointestinal bleeding, and should carry a card indicating that they are on anticoagulants in case of an accident. No other drugs should be taken simultaneously without medical advice.

Nursing action

The nurse will be involved in taking regular blood samples for prothrombin time estimation which is the guide to patient dosage. The usual prothrombin time is about 12 seconds and the dose should be adjusted to keep the level at about twice to three times normal. For the average patient on warfarin this normally means about 4–6 mg which can be taken in a single daily dose. Other anticoagulant measurements may be used by laboratories and the nurse should be familiar with the method used locally.

Once a patient is well controlled on anticoagulants the prothrombin time only needs to be estimated about once a month, but again, it is important that the patient realises the significance of attending regularly for blood tests and reporting any excessive bruising or bleeding (e.g. nose bleeds) between attendances.

Arthritis

The term arthritis is commonly used to mean osteoarthritis, an inflammatory reaction associated with age changes in the joints. However, rheumatoid arthritis has a quite different aetiology, although many of the drugs used in both conditions are similar.

General advice

Patients with stiff and swollen joints are often disabled and may need their morale boosting from time to time. The nurse will be involved in seeing these patients, both for blood tests and possibly for unrelated episodes of illness. She should always look for signs that the sufferer, particularly when elderly, is not becoming too depressed or isolated by his or her disability.

Some patients find that the nature of the weather makes a considerable difference to the symptoms, others that certain food-stuffs seem to make the joints more painful. Any approach which indicates that the doctor and the nurse care about the discomfort will help, and encouragement towards self-help and an independent existence is important.

The involvement or a domicillary physiotherapist or occupational therapist should always be considered in this respect.

Non-steroidal anti-inflammatory drugs (NSAIs)

This term covers a multitude of drugs now available, which claim to reduce inflammation, pain and swelling in inflammed joints. The group includes aspirin, ibuprofen (Brufen) and indomethacin (Indocid) which can be taken in doses of one or two tablets or capsules up to three times daily after food. There are some single dose preparations on the market, such as piroxicam (Feldene) which only need to be taken once daily.

All the drugs are effective to a greater or lesser extent in helping patients to cope with painful swollen joints and the doctor and the patient must discover the preparation which gives most relief without undue side-effects, particularly gastrointestinal, which may reduce the tolerance of the patient to using the drug. The use of the same drugs as suppositories (e.g. Indocid) sometimes overcomes these difficulties, and will aid morning stiffness if taken at night but can cause proctitis.

Steroids

The corticosteroid group of drugs are powerful and effective in many conditions, but have no place in osteoarthritis. There are many side-effects which include weight gain, gastric ulceration, reduced resist-ance to infection and osteoporosis. The patient should carry a card stating that he or she is on steroids and the dose being taken.

Steroids are dangerous because they reduce the ability of the patient's adrenal glands to respond to a crisis, such as an accident or severe infection, and the patient may go into profound 'adrenal shock' if this is not anticipated and treated by rapidly increasing the steroid dosage. Nevertheless, they are a useful group of drugs which have saved many lives, but the practice nurse should be aware of some of the problems of this group of drugs so that she can discuss them with the patient if the necessity arises.

Myocrisin and penicillamine

These drugs are of use in severe rheumatoid arthritis and myocrisin has to be given by injection. The nurse will be involved in this and usually a course of injections will be ordered. Penicillamine can be taken orally. However both drugs have major side-effects related to suppression of bone marrow, renal and liver damage and skin rashes. Because of this the nurse will regularly need to test the urine for albumen and take blood for biochemistry and screening for haemoglobin, red and white cell count and platelet count.

Asthma

Major developments have been made in the management of this condition over the last twenty years.

Bronchodilators

The commonly used drugs in this field are those blocking histamine receptors in the bronchi such as salbutamol (Ventolin) or similarly related substances, plus the long acting theophylline derivatives (e.g. Phyllocontin).

It is essential that the nurse knows the correct way to use an inhaler as they may have to instruct the patient. Many patients use inhalers incorrectly and squirt the contents into their mouth instead of correctly inhaling them. Figure 12.1 shows the correct way to use the inhaler. A patient who will benefit from an inhaler of this type will show a marked improvement on the Peak Flow Meter (see Chapter 6) before and after using it. Inhaled medication is preferable to oral as it reaches the receptor sites without using a large dose and with a consequent reduction in the risk of side effects.

The dose of salbutamol for an adult is about 4 mg of the tablets three times a day or two puffs of the inhaler three times daily or when necessary. A proportionally smaller dose for children is used and there is syrup with the normal dosage of 5 ml three times a day, although it is not suitable for children under two years old.

Administration of inhaled medication using a nebuliser is now common and the equipment is described in Chapter 6. It is particularly valuable for children.

The long-acting theophyllines are taken orally on a once or twice a day basis.

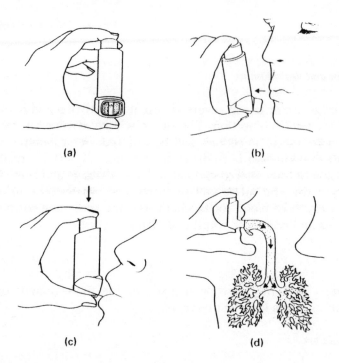

(a)   (b)

(c)   (d)

Fig. 12.1   How to use an inhaler. (a) Remove the cover from the mouthpiece. Hold the inhaler as illustrated and shake vigorously. (b) Breathe out slowly but no further than the end of a natural breath. (c) *Immediately* place the mouthpiece above the tongue and well into the mouth. Press the top of the cannister down firmly between forefinger and thumb whilst inhaling deeply and quickly. (d) Continue inhaling to carry the spray deep into the lungs. Hold the breath for as long as it is comfortable. Release pressure on the cannister, remove the inhaler from your mouth and breathe out *gently*.

Steroid inhalers

Steroids have always been useful in asthma but have the side effects and problems discussed earlier. A breakthrough occurred when a method of inhaling steroids was discovered which gave effective relief at much smaller doses than the oral preparations (e.g. Becotide).

The inhaled steroids can also be used with other inhalers such as salbutamol and the method of use is the same.

Sodium cromoglycate

This preparation is marketed as Intal and has a unique action in blocking the allergic response precipitating the asthmatic reaction before it occurs. It cannot be taken orally because of destruction in the gut. The manufacturers invented an interesting device called a spinhaler to get the powder into the patient's airway. A small propellor is rotated by the inhalation of the patient and propels the powder from the fractured capsule into the airway but it can now be used in an inhaler.

Similar preparations of sodium cromoglycate are used in eye drops for allergic conjunctivitis (Opticrom) and as an inhaler for nasal allergies (Rynacrom).

It is important that preparations containing steroids or sodium cromoglycate are used regularly, if they are to be of value, as they are of no use in an acute attack, unlike salbutamol. Patients must understand this difference, particularly since they are likely to be familiar with and taking a variety of preparations with different modes of action.

In the past few years there has been a rapid increase in a wide variety of simple methods of improving inhaler techniques. These include spacers and ventadisc. The nurse should familiarise herself with them and their correct usage if she is to play a key role in the management of the asthmatic patient (see Chapter 11).

Conjunctivitis

This is a common condition in general practice and the nurse who sees a patient with this condition must be certain that there is no foreign body or corneal ulcer underlying the reaction. In infective conjunctivitis, topical antibiotic drops such as chloramphenicol are used; in milder cases simple hygiene precautions and bathing the eyes with dilute saline or optrex will be sufficient. Allergic conjunctivitis can be treated using topical antihistamine drops.

There are many other preparations available for treating the eyes and the nurse's work is solely related to making sure that she is competent to examine and assess an eye to exclude a foreign body or ulcer. A full discussion of this will be found in Chapter 9.

Catarrh

A great many patients suffer from catarrh, some all the time (perennial rhinitis) and the majority only when suffering an acute upper respiratory infection.

The drugs used in treatment include the decongestive antihistamines and nasal drops such as ephedrine. The latter should not be used over a long period as they can permanently damage the nasal mucosa, but they do have a place in very short term management. Many over-the-counter preparations are available and the nurse should become familiar with a few so that she can advise patients appropriately.

General advice

The term catarrh covers a multitude of disorders related to the sensation of congestion in the nasal airways and sinuses. Because the causes are so varied the nurse must try and distinguish between the acute problem (e.g. a cold or hayfever) and the chronic situation (e.g. perennial rhinitis and chronic sinusitis). If simple over-the-counter remedies have already been tried, she should refer a patient with persistent symptoms to the doctor. In the case of obvious allergic causes she may give general advice about avoidance of known allergens such as animals, house dust or pollen.

Constipation

The attitude of patients to constipation tends not to be quite so obsessive as it used to be. However patients become anxious if their bowels do not work regularly and the consumption of the many tons of laxatives available bears witness to this. In general terms a patient should only be considered to be constipated when the bowels are more sluggish than normal for that person. The normal bowel habit may be several times a day in one person and once or twice a week in another. It is important to recognise that the normal range of bowel activity is very wide and not base advice only on personal experience.

The advice given will depend on the age group of the patient.

1   Babies often become constipated when their dietary intake is being changed, e.g. change from breast to bottle or milk to solids. Simple reassurance together with an increase in the amount of fluid given (not just milk) may be all that is required. Lactulose syrup is a mild hydrating agent which is effective in more stubborn cases.
2   Young children may be slow to acquire normal toilet training habits. This may be due to heredity, laziness or insufficient parental attention. Advice about toilet training can be given by a nurse or health visitor and it is important not to over emphasise bowel activities as too much attention focused on this normal activity can condition the child to be more conscious of its importance at any age.

Children also tend to be so absorbed in their daily activities that they forget to go to the toilet and become constipated in this way by suppressing the normal bowel reflexes. Usually these patients present with abdominal pain and the diagnosis is obvious, but if in doubt the doctor should be consulted. Simple laxatives such as lactulose syrup or magnesium hydroxide and liquid paraffin emulsion together with dietary advice is all that is required.

Dietary advice should be the same at any age. Roughage in the form of vegetables and fruit should be encouraged plus bran in the diet or as an additive in cereal.

There is no place for powerful purgatives in the management of constipation in children and rarely in adults.

3   Adults will have established their dietary and bowel habits. If constipation occurs then the dietary habits should be reviewed. Simple laxatives and modification of diet is normally all that is required. In refractory problems suppositories such as glycerine or stronger laxatives such as senna may be required. The risk of using powerful purgatives is that the patient becomes used to using them and the bowel becomes flaccid, losing its tone and reflexes and only functioning when stimulated by purgatives.

4   Elderly patients with constipation fall into two categories. Those who have always been sluggish can be treated as in **3**.

Constipation arising as a fresh symptom in a patient who has previously been regular should always be viewed with suspicion as it can be the early signs of significant bowel disease, especially diverticulitis or carcinoma. These patients should have a careful history taken especially enquiring about abdominal pain, weight loss and rectal bleeding. If these symptoms are present then the patient should be referred to the general practitioners and referral should take place anyway if constipation persists for more than a week or so.

Coughs

The medical profession is divided over the value of cough medicine in the management of patients with upper or lower respiratory symptoms. Pharmacologically there seems to be little evidence that cough linctus actually has any benefit, but patients often set great store by the medication prescribed by their doctor and this should not be forgotten. However, that is not to say that the doctor should accede to every request for cough linctus, and patients should be encouraged to purchase it for themselves if they feel they need it.

Marsh and his colleagues showed the dramatic decrease in workload in his northern practice which resulted when the partners took a decision to prescribe no more cough medicine.[1]

There are basically five types of cough medicine in terms of the action which they are supposed to have; if they are to be prescribed or recommended it is reasonable to try and identify the group most likely to be of help.

1   Pleasant, soothing syrup with little pharmacological component (e.g. simple linctus for children).
2   Cough suppressants. These are supposed to act by suppressing the cough reflex and contain codeine (e.g. linctus codeine or pholcodine).
3   Expectorants. By far the commonest group concerned belong to this category. They are supposed to encourage mucous to become more liquified by osmotic action within the lung tissue and consequently may actually make the cough worse (e.g. Benylin expectorant).
4   Antihistamines. On the assumption that many coughs are upper respiratory in nature and associated with catarrh, a vast number of proprietary preparations contain a mixture of anti-histamines in the hope that the patient's congested airways will be improved. The sedative side effects of this group should be remembered (e.g. phensedyl linctus).
5   Antispasmodics. Where wheeze is predominant in the symptoms the use of an antispasmodic to relieve the bronchoconstriction may be considered helpful. The commonly used antispasmodics, like salbutamol (Ventolin), can be given in syrup form or can be combined with other preparations (e.g. alupent expectorant which is a bronchodilator (orciprenaline) plus an expectorant).

Depression

The practice nurse is unlikely to have a great deal to do with the medication in depression as they need careful medical supervision, but she should know the basic principles behind them as she may be asked questions by the patient when she is seeing him or her for other reasons.

Most antidepressants prescribed in general practice belong to the tricyclic group (imipramine or amitriptyline) and there are many variations of these, some being slow release preparations which only need to be taken once a day. They have a number of features in common which the nurse should bear in mind.

1   They tend to be sedative and potentiate alcohol. The sedative effects are less marked the longer they are taken.
2   They are quickly lethal if taken in fairly small overdose especially with alcohol.
3   Any beneficial antidepressant effects are unlikely to be felt in much less than two or three weeks from starting treatment and patients

should be encouraged to persevere with treatment even if they are feeling no better (or even worse!).

4   They may have other side effects such as blurred vision or dry mouth which may cause the patient to stop taking them.

There is another group of antidepressants called the monoamine oxidase inhibitors (MAOI). These are used in certain types of depression and phobic states and great care needs to be exercised with this group as they interact with many other drugs and foodstuffs. All patients on MAOIs must be warned of this and given written instructions stating:

(a)   the drug should be used with care
(b)   that no other drugs, including aspirin, should be taken without the permission of their doctor
(c)   that foodstuffs containing tyramine will react with the MAOIs to produce a severe rise in blood pressure. These foods include cheese, Bovril and Marmite.

Lithium is used in patients suffering from manic depressive psychosis and blood levels of the drug need to be taken regularly to adjust the dose if it is approaching the toxic level.

Diabetes

The practice nurse may well be more associated with these patients over a long period of time than any other group and will have an active part to play in their long term care. She will give advice about injection techniques and urine testing when they are first diagnosed, and may see them regularly for weight checks and dietary advice. These aspects are discussed in Chapter 11.

Diabetics fall into three categories:

1   Those dependent upon insulin.
2   Those who can manage with oral hypoglycaemic drugs.
3   Those who can be controlled on diet alone.

Insulin-dependent diabetics

Basically the insulins used are either short acting (soluble insulin, actrapid) or long acting (lente and ultratard) and the patient should be stabilised on one or a mixture of these.

All insulin strengths were standardised to U100 insulin with 100 units in 1 millilitre in 1984 and all patients previously on other insulins should be familiar with the new ones. New syringes have been issued with graduation to 100 units in each millilitre and this should reduce the confusion caused by the previous 20, 40 and 80 units/ml ampoules which have now been phased out.

The short acting insulins produce their maximum effect in about two or three hours from the time of the injection and the long acting ones some eight or ten hours after injection. It is important to know this when explaining hypoglycaemic reactions to patients.

Oral hypoglycaemic agents

Older patients develop diabetes when their pancreatic function starts to fail and the oral hypoglycaemic preparations (e.g. tolbutamide or glibenclamide) act by stimulating the remaining insulin secreting cells to perform more efficiently (i.e. by encouraging the patient's own biochemistry to deal more efficiently with his or her metabolism).

Obviously, if they are suitable for a patient, it is preferable to take tablets than have a daily injection and severe hypoglycaemic reactions are much less common. They do have other side effects such as skin rashes which may reduce their value in a particular patient and occasionally severe metabolic effects.

The routine management of diabetic patients in general practice is discussed fully in Chapter 11.

Diarrhoea

Diarrhoea is a common condition, but the nurse should always remember that this simple complaint may mask more serious conditions and that young babies are at risk of rapid dehydration. Remember also that in young children gastrointestinal symptoms may be due to upper respiratory infection.

The best treatment for acute symptoms likely to be associated with a simple gastrointestinal infection or dietary indiscretion is starvation with fluids only, and any prescribed treatment is of no value if this advice is not given. Antibiotics have no part to play, even in salmonella infections, and may exacerbate the symptoms. Kaolin or kaolin and morphine mixtures are available without prescription and can be used to settle the bowel in doses of 10–15 ml four times a day. Other preparations such as codeine phosphate, diphenoxylate and atropine (Lomotil) or loperamide (Imodium) may be prescribed if the symptoms are unduly prolonged or severe. No patient with severe diarrhoea should go for more than 24 hours without seeking medical advice, and children under one year of age should always be seen by a doctor at the onset of symptoms.

General advice

The practice nurse will be asked to provide advice to patients with gastrointestinal symptoms either by telephone or when seen on the practice premises. It is very difficult to assess the severity of symptoms of a patient by telephone and if in doubt the patient must be seen by a doctor. This is particularly true for young children or anyone with severe abdominal pain.

The commonest mistake made by patients in management is to start a normal dietary intake too quickly and not allow the bowel an adequate recovery time. Fluids should first be only water and/or fruit juices, going on to other fluids such as diluted milk and soup as symptoms subside and only returning to a completely normal diet over the course of about two days. Very young children can be provided with an electrolyte fluid drink (Dioralyte) to compensate for fluid loss, and when bottle feeding quarter, half and full strength milk should be returned to in that order. In bottle fed children a review of the sterilising procedure used by the mother should exclude faulty technique.

Eczema

The terms eczema and dermatitis are esentially the same and mean an inflammatory condition of the skin. Eczema may be due to a number of causes but the treatments are often the same. In mild inflammatory conditions simple calamine may be sufficient to help the symptoms. If the rash is weeping then set preparations such as potassium permanganate soaks will help to dry it. The commoner treatments, however, lie in the many different brands of steroid ointment and cream preparations available. They are very effective but not without their own problems if used over a long period of time. One of the most serious long-term effects is the loss of elasticity and thinning of the skin which occurs and is not reversible. In addition they often contain additives such as neomycin which may sensitise the skin and aggravate rather than cure the condition.

General advice

The nurse's main role will be to give simple advice on skin care and to refer patients back for assessment to the doctor if she finds they have been using a preparation for a long time without adequate supervision. Skin care includes advice about wearing suitable materials. Many man-made fibres cause allergic reactions. Contact eczema of the hands caused by washing powders can be helped by wearing rubber gloves, especially if a cotton glove is worn inside the rubber one, as some people are also sensitive to rubber.

People who suffer from eczema should avoid scented soaps and use simple baby soaps and in addition avoid scented talcum powder or other potential skin irritants (e.g. foaming bath salts).

Epilepsy

There are many new drugs on the market now for the management of epilepsy and phenobarbitone should no longer have to be prescribed. There is little point in stopping the drug in those patients who have been on it for many years, but no new patient should have it prescribed if other, less addictive and more effective, drugs are available. Currently used drugs include phenytoin (Epanutin), carbamazepine (Tegretol) and sodium valproate (Epilim).

It is usual to monitor the blood levels of these drugs because it is important to adjust them to the individual needs, and the toxic and therapeutic range is close. The nurse will do this and is responsible for entering both the time of the last dose of the drug and the time the sample was taken on the laboratory request form, because both are required in assessing the result. (See Chapter 5 Table 5.1.)

Whenever the nurse sees the patient she should check that he or she is taking the drug regularly and enquire about any side effects, such as drowsiness. Phenytoin causes an unpleasant hypertrophic reaction of the gums and folate deficiency in some people.

Heart failure

The term heart failure describes the results of failing efficiency of the right or left side of the heart or a combination of both. The patient commonly complains of breathlessness and swollen ankles and is usually elderly or has a history of cardiac problems. Many drugs are used to manage this condition, but treatment is essentially dependent upon diuretics and the cardiac glycosides (digoxin).

Digoxin (Lanoxin)

Digoxin has been in use for centuries and was frequently overprescribed. It acts by making the myocardium more efficient in its contraction and so increases cardiac output. The blood level can be monitored; the first signs of digoxin toxicity are a bradycardia with a fall of the pulse rate below 60 per minute, together with nausea.

Diuretics

The diuretics are a group of drugs with many different actions and uses but essentially they all act by reducing the amount of oedema found in excess in the lungs or other tissues as in heart failure. They have a direct action on the kidneys and so a consequence of use is that the patient will pass more urine and they should be warned of this. Examples of diuretics are bendrofluazide (Navidrex), frusemide (Lasix) and spironolactone (Aldactone). They are usually taken as a morning dose so that diuresis does not disturb the sleep. Due to osmolarity changes in the kidneys produced by the action of some diuretics there may be a loss of significant amounts of potassium, which may be replaced by giving a potassium supplement. If supplements are not given patients should be encouraged to eat fruit with a high potassium content, such as bananas or oranges.

Hypertension

The long-term effects of uncontrolled high blood pressure on the patient are now well recognised and a large number of products are available to reduce the systolic and diastolic levels to more acceptable readings.

Most medication in asymptomatic patients tends to make them feel 'slowed up' or worse than they felt when untreated. This means that patients may cease to take their medication, or not take it regularly, if they do not understand the reasons behind the treatment.

The practice nurse will be involved when she takes the patient's blood pressure at routine checks or because the practice has a policy of routinely recording the blood pressure levels of all the patients as described in Chapter 11.

What is 'the normal blood pressure' is open to debate. Some authorities would maintain that all middle-aged patients with a persistent level about 140/90 should be treated and others would accept higher figures. No patient should be diagnosed as hypertensive on one isolated reading, but the reading should be repeated on several occasions after rest and lying down before a final decision is made. It is as well to remember that the diagnosis of hypertension commits the patient and the doctor to a lifetime of medication and supervision and this should not be undertaken lightly.

There are many groups of drugs used in treating hypertension, including the beta blockers (e.g. atenolol), the peripheral vasodilators (e.g. prazosin) and the group of ACE inhibitors (e.g. captopril). The nurse need not concern herself with details of action but should use her influence to encourage the patient to take the drugs as prescribed and to report side effects.

Indigestion

Probably more over-the-counter remedies are bought for indigestion than for most other symptoms. The majority of causes are usually self-evident and often associated with factors such as poor eating habits, heavy smoking or high alcohol consumption. Again, prescribing without an assessment of the causes is valueless.

Antacids

Antacids are effective in relieving many gastrointestinal symptoms. Commonly used antacids include aluminium hydroxide (Aludrox) and a mixture of magnesium trisilicate. They should be taken after or between meals, and often an extra dose at bedtime or in the night soothes the symptoms of gastritis or peptic ulceration. There is little difference between liquid preparations and tablets; those at work may prefer tablets for convenience.

H_2 receptor antagonist

In recent years a totally new type of preparation has come on the market. It was found that cimetidine (Tagamet) and, later, ranitidine (Zantac) selectively blocked the acid-secreting cells in the gastric mucosa so that there was a considerable reduction in acid production; this had a dramatic effect on the healing of gastric ulcers. It may have some beneficial effect on duodenal ulcers, too. These preparations should be prescribed for a specific course of several weeks, and then a maintenance dose supervised medically as the long term effects of taking these are not yet known and the preparation is moderately expensive.

Antiflatulence

Patients often complain of a bloated feeling in association with other gastrointestinal symptoms and some preparations are designed to each absorb excess air in the bowel such as Asilone or actually to break down large pockets of air into bubbles (Gaviscon). Both of these are proprietary mixtures of various antacids such as aluminium hydroxide and other constituents, e.g. dimethicone or alginic acid.

It should be emphasised that indigestion as a symptom can mask many serious problems and no patient should take antacids or other similar preparations for long periods of time without seeking medical advice. The nurse may be the first person consulted and she should see that any patient taking antacids regularly, having a lot of pain or loss of weight is referred to the doctor.

Infections

Probably the most overused and overprescribed group of drugs in general practice are the antibiotics. These are often prescribed for viral conditions in which they have no effect or may be expected by patients who have been led to believe that they are a panacea for all ills.

Antibiotics

There are many different antibiotics available and they are only of value in specific infections. Unfortunately, it is not always possible to be certain whether an infection is bacterial or viral but doctors must use their clinical judgement in this respect and not, for example, prescribe an antibiotic routinely in all patients with a sore throat.

Antibiotics basically fall into two groups—bacteriocidal (e.g. penicillin) and bacteriostatic (e.g. tetracycline). The first actually kills the infecting organism and the second inhibits its growth while the normal defence mechanisms of the body overcome the infection.

The simple and older antibiotics such as penicillin tend not to be used as much since broad spectrum, more impressive-looking tablets and capsules have been developed. However, penicillin and tetracycline are still very effective and often do not have the side effects of the more powerful antibiotics. Broad spectrum refers to the range of organisms against which the drug is effective. Tetracycline should not be given in children because of the absorption into developing teeth with consequent effects on the dentition. The teeth are mottled and often distorted in these cases. Previous known sensitivity reaction to an antibiotic should be borne in mind when prescribing them and the records should clearly draw attention to this.

Medical personnel must emphasise to the patient the importance of taking the full course of treatment prescribed and to report back if a rash or gastrointestinal side effects develop. Many patients do not complete a course of antibiotics because they forgot, misread or misunderstood the correct dosage, or got better before completing the course of treatment. The newer once and twice daily preparations may improve patient compliance but are relatively more expensive for the NHS than the same type of antibiotic taken more frequently.

Topically applied antibiotics are of use in superficial skin infections such as impetigo, but care must be taken because patients may develop skin sensitivity to topically applied antibiotics, particularly neomycin.

Antiseptic solutions

For local infection on the skin, bathing with a simple antiseptic solution is often sufficient (e.g. TCP, Savlon and eusol). Other local applications are discussed in Chapter 5.

Mouthwashes are sometimes used and may be recommended by the practice nurse. Simple salt water mouthwash (one teaspoonful of salt in a tumbler of warm water) is very useful after dental extraction or severe tonsillitis. Other mouthwashes include Oraldene, TCP or hydrogen peroxide.

Insomnia

Doctors are often requested by patients to prescribe something to 'help them sleep'. Certainly the consumption of hypnotics of one sort or another has become commonplace.

A great deal is now known about the nature of sleep and the way in which the various drugs prescribed affect it. Many patients have a high expectation of a perfect night's sleep and eight hours of refreshing unconsciousness each night, irrespective of age, other concomitant illness or their own personal needs.

The nurse may have an opportunity to advise patients who are having difficulty in sleeping. They should be reassured that everyone has periods of disturbed sleep and that as one grows older the amount of continuous sleep required is reduced. If an elderly patient has several short naps during the day they will not sleep so well at night and indeed do not require to do so. If the expectation can be changed patients may come to terms with their sleep pattern.

Warm milk drinks, a hot bath and reading in bed before settling for sleep all encourage the mind and body to wind down from the day's activities. Barbiturates should *never* be prescribed in new cases as many patients are still addicted to those which were dispensed over twenty years ago by doctors before the problems were realised. Many hypnotics have mildly addictive and habituation problems anyway and should be prescribed with care and supervised regularly, e.g. nitrazepam (Mogadon), temazepam (Normison) or flurazepam (Dalmane) and the hazards of benzodiazepines to which these all belong are well recognised.

Migraine

Headaches are often labelled as migraine when not presenting the typical picture. The true migraine headache is unilateral, often associated with visual disturbance and vomiting, may be associated with certain foods or stress, and often genetic in origin. It is due to sudden and unilateral dilation of the cerebral vessels. Treatment includes rest in a dark room, avoidance of precipitating factors and general advice about the nature of the condition. If attacks are not severe then simple analgesics such as paracetamol or codeine may suffice. If nausea and vomiting are prominent features then pro-chlorperazine (Stemetil) is often useful as are other drugs of a similar nature.

Specific treatment lies with the ergotamine group of drugs which will only relieve the true migraine headache. The commonest example of this is Migril. All of this group must be taken with care and the stated dose not exceeded as ergotamine has vasospastic effects on the peripheral circulation and can cause gangrene if taken in overdosage.

Proprietary preparations, such as Migraleve, can be purchased from the chemist and some patients find these helpful.

Pain

Perhaps the group of drugs about which the nurse will most often be asked is those which relieve pain. In recent years the traditional aspirin and paracetamol have come under attack in the medical press, aspirin because it can cause acute gastric erosion with bleeding, and parace-tamol because it is toxic to the liver in overdose. This should not prevent one from encouraging patients to use their commonsense when wishing to take something for pain. If the medication is taken with at least half a glass of water or milk gastrointestinal problems are reduced.

Aspirin

Because of the gastrointestinal side effects, this is better taken in the soluble form or with food. It is effective as an analgesic, anti-inflammatory and antipyretic and therefore still has a part to play in febrile illness. It is not recommended for children below the age of 12 years.

Paracetamol

Paracetamol has similar effects to aspirin but does not cause the gastrointestinal problems. Moderation must be advised since overdos-age will cause hepatocellular damage. The soluble preparations are valuable in children.

Codeine

This is a stronger analgesic which is often combined with aspirin or paracetamol (e.g. Panadeine) and tends to be constipating. Its allied compound dihydrocodeine (DF 118) is a very effective analgesic and in oral form is not classified as a controlled drug.

Coproxamol (Distalgesic)

This preparation has been in use as a moderately strong analgesic for a long time and is a combination of paracetamol and dextropropoxyphene. Again, it has become unpopular because with alcohol it can be lethal since a small overdose will produce severe CNS effects. However, it would seem a pity to deprive patients of its benefits if overdose is not a risk and it has widespread use in musculoskeletal conditions.

The opiates

Regulations concerning the use of this group of drugs is discussed in Chapter 13 and the nurse is not likely to be asked by patients about them. She may have responsibility for the drug cupboard and the keeping up of the dangerous drug register in some practices.

Schizophrenia

The management of severe psychiatric illness has changed dramatically in the past twenty years with the introduction of powerful drugs, and the policy of keeping psychiatric patients in the community whenever possible. The practice nurse will increasingly have contact with patients suffering from schizophrenia since many are prescribed a long-acting depot injection preparation of phenothiazine drugs. The side effects of this group are Parkinson-like tremor, and she should be aware of this as the patient may require extra medication to treat this if it develops or the dose modified. It is also important to know if these patients are defaulting from their weekly or two-weekly injections and she should keep a recall register (see Chapter 3) to monitor their attendance.

These patients can be unpredictable in their behaviour and the nurse should try and avoid being alone with them.

Stress

Modern society seems increasingly to place its members under stress and the use of tranquillisers has rocketed in the last twenty years. The risks of chronic habituation from taking these drugs is now realised and given widespread publicity so that patients are becoming more willing to face life without drug support; nevertheless, the numbers of tranquillisers being consumed is vast. Doctors must try and resist inappropriate demands for this type of support and encourage their patients to manage without them.

Most of this group belong to the benzodiazepines, of which the most popular is diazepam (Valium). They are all sedatives to a greater or lesser extent and their effects are potentiated in the presence of alcohol. Consequently, patients should be warned of this so that care is taken when driving.

Patients should be encouraged to take responsibility for coping with stress in ways which do not involve drug dependence, be it smoking, alcohol or tranquillisers, and the nurse will have a specific part to play in counselling these patients when she sees them. Yoga, relaxation classes and hypnotherapy all have a part to play in reducing the tensions of anxious patients. Advice may have to be given about working conditions together with counselling about realistic life goals.

Urinary tract infection

Adults

The complaint of cystitis is very common in women and may mean anything from pyelonephritis to a little pain on micturation. The significance from the nurse's point of view is that these problems are very common and may or may not be associated with proven urinary tract infection. The nurse will be involved in collecting mid-stream urine samples (MSUs) for culture and possibly other samples, such as urethral and vaginal swabs. Treatment may need to be prolonged in refractory cases and it is important for the nurse to check that the patient is taking the medication correctly and that repeat MSUs are collected as specified by the doctor.

The actual treatment is usually an antibiotic which may be broad spectrum, (e.g. ampicillin) or a specific urinary tract one (e.g. nitrofurantoin). The urinary tract antibiotics are chosen because a high proportion of the preparation is excreted through the kidneys and reaches satisfactory treatment levels in the urine. Some doctors may use a two or three day course of treatment with a large dose of medication, but the common method is about ten days of antibiotics. It is desirable that an MSU is checked before commencing treatment and a further one checked a few days after completing the course to confirm that the causative organism has been eradicated.

For women who suffer from transitory urethral or bladder symptoms after intercourse an MSU often does not culture an organism, and all that may be required is a few doses of mist potassium citrate to alkalise the urine which kills off the transient bacteruria.

Children

The situation in children is quite different. Undiagnosed urinary infection in childhood can lead to a low grade chronic pyelonephritis with no symptoms, which in adult life leads ultimately to renal failure. It is vital, therefore, that the urine of children (especially girls) be examined if there is the slightest chance of a urinary infection being present.

Treatment is by using antibiotics but in this case they may need to be taken for a prolonged period, up to several years, with repeated MSUs about every three months. These children are usually found on investigation to have reflux of urine up the ureters on micturition, due to inefficient development of the valves at the ureto bladder junction. If they can be kept free of infection the majority develop the use of these valves at about eight to ten years old, and can then come off all treatment. The nurse, therefore, has a major role to play in taking samples from these children and encouraging the parents to attend regularly for follow-up. She will also check that the medication is being taken and emphasise the good long term prognosis if management is followed properly.

General advice

The nurse has a major role to play in the management of urinary infections in general practice. She will be responsible for collecting, storing and dispatching MSU specimens which, if incorrectly collected, may be contaminated, or if not stored properly will give false negative results, because the organisms will have died by the time the sample reaches the laboratory. In positive cases it is important to ensure that the patient has follow-up samples taken and, as already explained, the nurse has long term responsibility for supervising children under treatment.

Women can often reduce the frequency of their attacks of cystitis by simple remedies and it is important to give these women the following instructions.

1   Pay careful attention to perineal toilet. Toilet paper should be

wiped from front to back to reduce the chances of bringing organisms into contact with the genitourinary system.

2   Keep up a moderately high fluid intake and pass water immediately after intercourse.

3   Try and avoid restrictive clothing, especially tights.

Many patient advice leaflets are available and an example is given in Appendix X.

Vaginal discharge

Many women have varying amounts of vaginal discharge present, either at certain times of the menstrual cycle or all the time. It is important to establish exactly what a woman is complaining about when she says she has a vaginal discharge.

The commonest infective causes of this symptom are vaginal monilia (candidiasis), trichomonas and chlamydia.

Candida

Women taking oral contraceptives or those who are pregnant are more likely to get a fungal infection as candida is a normal inhabitant of the skin and the resistance of the vaginal mucosa to infection is reduced in these conditions. The discharge is thick and cheesy and very irritating. Treatment is simple and consists of using a variety of antifungal agents such as clotrimazole (Canesten), Nystatin or miconazole (Gyno-daktarin) as pessaries and topical applications. The partner should be treated even if asymptomatic to prevent reinfection.

Trichomonas vaginalis

Trichomonas vaginalis is a venereal disease as it is transmitted by intercourse. The causative agent is a flagellate organism and is effectively treated by metronidazole (Flagyl) taken orally for a week.

Chlamydia

Chlamydia, another protozoa, is increasingly being recognised as a common cause of resistant vaginal discharge or pelvic inflammatory disease. It can only be identified if swabs are taken carefully (Chapter 5) and responds to treatment with oxytetracycline.

General advice

There are other causes of vaginal discharge but the nurse's role is confined to taking vaginal swabs if she has been taught to do so and giving advice to the patient. This may be general advice about hygiene or sexual activities. The opportunity should never be lost to offer contraceptive advice if this seems appropriate and to reassure patients that vaginal infections are common and treatable if instructions are followed.

When collecting samples do not forget that more than one infection may be present, in particular, it is difficult clinically to diagnose gonorrhoea in women, therefore swabs should be taken with the greatest care if this organism is not to be missed.

Recurrent monilial infection is a particular problem for some women and they may need advice about changing their oral contraception, general hygiene and the wearing of tights which seems to predispose to this condition.

Warts

Warts are caused by a virus and can present as lesions on the fingers, body, feet (verruca) or genital and anal region. The treatment is essentially the same for all and as effective (or ineffective!) in any site. Warts have a high rate of recurrence which is why it is sometimes difficult to deal with them satisfactorily. An assortment of topical applications may be used such as podophyllin, formaldehyde and glutaraldehyde (Glutarol). They act by inhibiting the growth of the wart and care should be taken to protect the normal surrounding skin from damage.

General advice

Warts on the fingers can be treated with podophyllin preparations. The patient should put some vaseline on the surrounding skin to protect it and then podophyllin ointment or paint applied to the wart. The wart should then be covered with an elastoplast and the procedure repeated each day. The skin may become white, soggy and sore and if this is severe the patient should stop treatment for several days and leave it uncovered until it settles down. Treatment usually has to continue for several weeks and recommenced at the first sign of recurrence.

Plantar warts (verrucae) cause a great deal of consternation at schools and swimming baths and many children are deprived unnecessarily of school sporting and swimming activities. The verruca is usually acquired in showers or changing room but, provided an elastoplast dressing and footware are used, except when actually swimming, the chance of cross-infection is slight. Daily topical application of glutaraldehyde (Glutarol) is usually effective and the wart should be scraped each night to remove dead skin before the next application. Treatment is usually prolonged and several weeks of application will be required for success.

Genital warts are sexually transmitted and can spread rapidly in the damp warm conditions ideal for their propagation. Topical treatment with podophyllin or liquid nitrogen is effective but great care has to be taken not to overtreat the genital area. They are often associated with other sexually transmitted disease and it is recommended that patients should be referred to the hospital special clinic so that they can be screened for these (including HIV status) and their partner also traced.

Surgery

Some doctors prefer to surgically remove warts either by curretting them out or cauterising them. There is no indication that this is more or less successful in preventing recurrences than the more time-consuming topical applications. However, refractory warts are probably best tackled in this way and the nurse will be responsible for laying out the trolley and assisting the doctor.

Try and resist parental pressure to have verrucae treated in this way as it is unnecessarily traumatic for the child and resistant ones are better treated with liquid nitrogen.

REFERENCES

1   Day J. (1986) *Diabetic Handbook*. Diabetic Association.

Chapter 13

The Practice Nurse and the Law

The practice nurse will be involved legally with two different types of situation as a result of working in the treatment room. The first is her professional liability as a nurse treating patients, the second is her responsibilities as an employee in the practice. These two aspects have quite different implications and will be dealt with separately.

PROFESSIONAL LIABILITIES

There has been a significant change in the disciplinary structure of the nursing profession. On the 1st July 1983 the General Nursing Council and another eight professional and training bodies were abolished and replaced by the United Kingdom Central Council for Nursing, Midwifery and Health Visiting (UKCC). There are four national boards of the UKCC for England, Scotland, Wales and Northern Ireland.

The statutory disciplinary function of the GNC has now been replaced by a system of investigating committees. These committees will consider the evidence presented in a complaints procedure and may 'advise' the nurse concerned, or refer the matter to the UKCC professional conduct committee for further action. A professional conduct guide issued by the UKCC states a number of guidelines for professional behaviour.

1 Compliance with the law of the land in which he or she works.
2 Accountability for his or her practice as a nurse.
3 Regard for the customs and beliefs of the patients.
4 Confidentiality of patient information.
5 No abuse of the privileged relationship with patients.
6 Promote the safety and well being of patients under his or her care.
7 Regard to the environment of care and reference to the appropriate authority if this endangers safe standards of practice.

8   Responsibility to less experienced peers and subordinates to develop professional competence.
9   Take action on workload pressures if these endanger safe standards of practice.
10 Notifying the relevant authority of any conscientious objection which he or she may hold relevant to professional practice.
11 Refuse to accept gifts or favours which might be interpreted as exerting undue influence to obtain preferential treatment.
12 Avoid advertising.

The role of the practice nurse has developed gradually and it has already been implied in this book that many nurses and doctors are still not exactly sure of their individual role in those grey areas in which responsibilities overlap. Examples of these grey areas include syringing of ears, giving immunisations and assessing patients who have presented themselves to the nurse without first seeing a doctor.

Although the situation is somewhat confused there are a number of guidelines which do seem to help when considering this difficult problem.

1   The practice nurse is a professional person with her own professional liability for her actions.
2   She is employed by either a general practitioner or a health authority; the employer also has a legal responsibility. This is a vicarious liability in law and may result in a patient making a claim against the employer rather than the individual nurse.
3   Whoever is responsible for the liability, there is no doubt that if a nurse undertakes an activity for which she has not been properly trained, there really is no defence in law.

   The training may take the form of general professional nursing training, specific extra training (e.g. family planning) or the nurse may be trained to do a particular task by her employer. Evidence would have to be produced to show that the nurse had adequate training and that it was reasonable for the employer to expect her to carry out a particular task competently.
4   The nurse's legal protection is much higher if she is a member of a professional body such as the Royal College of Nursing. This body will also be able to give her specific advice on an individual problem if she wishes it.
5   No doctor should employ a practice nurse who does not have some form of professional liability cover and, of course, the doctor also needs to have his or her professional defence union membership. There are some insurance companies who will cover a nurse for professional claims without a professional society but this should be the minimum legal protection that a practice nurse should have.

These five principles can be used as a guide in trying to define professional liability in a given situation. Some simple examples might make the matter clearer.

(a)   A nurse gives an injection of iron for which the patient has been seen by the doctor and a prescription issued. While giving the injection the needle breaks and the patient makes a claim. In this case the nurse would be liable as giving injections is clearly seen as a nursing task for which she will have been trained.

(b)   A nurse has worked previously in a casualty department and was trained there to suture minor wounds. Her GP employer supervises her in this activity on a few occasions when she first comes into his employment. She then sutures a simple wound on the arm which becomes secondarily infected, breaks down and leaves a scar. The patient makes a claim. In this case there might well be no liability on either nurse or doctor as she could be shown to have been trained to undertake a task which was within her competence. The fact that a secondary problem arose was not her fault unless she had not treated the condition correctly in the first place.

(c)   A patient complaining of abdominal pain is seen by the nurse and sent home without referral to the doctor. Later that night the patient perforates an inflamed appendix and eventually makes a claim. In this case it would be considered as a vicarious liability of the general practitioner employer on the grounds of the employer's legal liability for his or her employee's negligent decision.

While these three cases are fairly straightforward no doubt the legal profession could still produce arguments for or against various actions. It is important for the nurse to be aware of her professional responsibilities, but to act in the best interests of the patient, in which case she is not likely to have much to fear. Unfortunately, in these litigation-conscious days everyone is at risk of being taken to court for any number of reasons.

The Medicine Act (1968)

The Medicine Act (1968) states that only certain named persons can be designated as prescribers of prescription-only medicines. The designated persons are doctors, dentists and veterinary surgeons, and all vaccines are included in this list (Medicines Order 1980).

The Royal College of Nursing goes to great lengths to point out to practice nurses that they are not exempt from this Act and should not give patients vaccines without specific *written* instructions to do so from the doctor. It does not need to be a formal prescription on an FP10 form, but for substances which are often kept in stock it could be an instruction in the patient's medical record.

A written prescription is different from the general written instruction. The general written instruction authorises occupational health nurses to obtain and administer prescription-only medicines specified to persons in general who may be in need of treatment. In this case the doctor can identify the drugs to be used and the circumstances under which their use is authorised. It is the nurse's responsibility to decide how and when and to whom these general written instructions apply. However, practice nurses are not occupational health nurses, although this might be seen as an area for professional negotiators to consider.

Repeat instructions included in the original prescription can be followed without reference back to the doctor.

If a prescription for an injection or vaccine is being given on the written instruction of the doctor it is no excuse for the nurse to give this if contraindications exist. She must not assume that the doctor is aware of the contraindication to a particular injection, even if the prescription is written, without checking herself that a contraindication does not exist before she gives the injection.

It is also the nurse's professional responsibility to keep up-to-date on techniques and changes in current thinking. As a result of being out-of-date professionally and therefore not showing sufficient care in a specific action, she may be held negligent. Obviously the patient or those legally responsible for the patient must give consent before a course of treatment is given, thus that the patient presents or is presented for the injection is implied consent.

Chapter 3 of this book was devoted to record systems and this just serves to illustrate the importance of all members of the primary health care team keeping adequate records.

There are differences of opinion about the question of whether the Royal College of Nursing is correct in interpreting the Medicine Act (1968) to mean that 'the prescription must exist first'. Dr Garth Hill of the Medical Defence Union, in reply to a question on this subject, stated that in their solicitor's opinion if the patient referred to is a patient of the doctor for whom the nurse is working, then there is nothing illegal in giving a direction to a practice nurse to immunise those patients. Anyone (it need not be a nurse) can administer a medicine under the direction of a doctor.

The Royal College of Nursing has issued an important booklet entitled, 'Drug Administration—A Nursing Responsibility', and all nurses should read this. It covers such items as professional responsibility in relation to drugs and their administration. Although it is directed at hospital and community nurses the principles apply equally for the practice nurse.

The issue of whether or not a prescription has to be written before a drug or vaccine can be administered will probably exercise the medical and nursing professions for some time to come. In most cases the situation will be quite clear and drugs will be prescribed and given. In some cases, the question is still in doubt for routine administration of an item such as a vaccine to a registered patient of the practice, where this is the standard procedure for the practice and no contraindications arise. Finally, even the Royal College of Nursing agrees that there are such emergency situations (e.g. anaphylactic shock) where a drug may have to be given by a nurse when no doctor is available to issue a prescription.

It cannot be emphasised too often that full documentation on drugs or vaccines given to a patient must be recorded on the patient's notes. This is particularly important for nurses working on their own as they do not have the security of a double check on drugs before administration such as occurs in normal hospital routine.

CONDITIONS OF EMPLOYMENT

Legal responsibilities for employers and employees in regard to their work place are different from the professional liabilities discussed earlier in the chapter.

There are a number of different issues and Acts of Parliament involved which overlap in some areas. These relate to employees or patients injured, in this case on practice premises, and are:

Occupiers Liability Act 1957
Employers Liability (Defective Equipment) Act 1969
Consumer Protection Act 1987
Health and Safety at Work Act 1974
Factory Acts, Office, Shops and Railway Premises Act and other Statutes and Regulations

Occupiers Liability Act 1957

Any occupier of premises has a duty in relation to the care of those premises and may be liable if negligence can be proved. The premises may be privately owned by the GP or be owned by the health authority.

In the simple example of a nurse (or patient) tripping on a defective step and injuring themselves the occupier of the premises would be liable for not attending to the repair of that step and be also liable under the Health and Safety at Work Act for not taking reasonable care to attend to the safety of employees. In the terms of the Act an occupier is anyone who can be said to be in control of those premises at the time of the accident.

Employers Liability (Defective Equipment) Act 1969

If an employee or patient is injured by faulty equipment, for example, being cut by breaking glass or given a severe shock by faulty electrical equipment, then the employer may be at fault through vicarious liability for not insuring the safety of his equipment. However, if all reasonable care had been taken and it could be proved that the equipment itself was faulty then the manufacturers or suppliers might be at fault. In this case the employee could claim compensation from the employer who would then make out a case against the supplier or manufacturer concerned.

As from 1988 in the case quoted above a 'no fault' claim may be possible under the Consumer Protection Act. In this case if the manufacturer can show that in the light of manufacturing development at the time that the equipment was found to be faulty the defect was not such that other similar producers would be expected to have discovered the defect in their own products. A defect is widely defined in the terms of the Act and may be no more than the safety of the product was not such that persons generally are entitled to expect.

Violence in the surgery

A regrettable trend of the last few years has been the increasing number of attacks by patients or others on the medical and nursing profession.

If the practice nurse is injured on the premises by a violent patient she has a number of actions which she can take.

1 Sue the person concerned in the criminal courts.
2 Sue the employer for his vicarious liability in being negligent in protecting her. In this case it would have to be demonstrated that the practice or the health authority had not taken reasonable precautions to protect the nurse from potentially violent patients. For example, it might be appropriate to have an alarm system in the treatment room or for nurses to be warned in advance about potentially violent patients e.g. mentally disturbed patients attending for treatment.
3 Even if no liability can be claimed it is sometimes possible to obtain compensation from the Criminal Injuries Compensation Board although the process is tedious and the rewards likely to be small.

The whole area of employers and employees liability is a complex one and the examples given above are only relatively simple ones. A number of helpful articles are now appearing in the nursing publications and if there is any doubt about the legal liabilities of the practice both as employers and for the employees then expert advice should be sought.

It is important that nurses are familiar with their rights under the terms of the various employment acts. They should also bear in mind that if they are part-time, then the fewer rights they have and that when they are employed for less than eight hours a week, to all intents and purposes they have no rights in terms of notice and dismissal.

There are no specific rates of pay for practice nurses employed by GPs, but the Royal College of Nursing recommends that they have comparable responsibility with a Ward Sister and that they should be paid at this rate or the current Whitley Pay Grade, depending on experience and incremental rises. This assumes that the nurse is State Registered or Registered General. If she is State Enrolled General then she should be paid on the current scale, depending on experience and incremental rises.

A new grading scale was recommended in 1988 by the Royal College of Nursing and on this scale practice nurses would be in grade G (post basic qualifications, DNC, OHNC, HV cert etc.) or Grade H. The new Grade H is an interesting development and to qualify for this scale the nurse should provide clinical advice/support to the extended primary health care team and have responsibilities for developing practice clinical policies as well as being involved in at least three of the following criteria:

(a)   Teaching other practice nurses.
(b)   Controlling admission to her own list.
(c)   Carrying out and interpreting certain tests.
(d)   Buying practice equipment.
(e)   Initiating and carrying out research.
(f)   Managing the nursing team.
(g)   Controlling resources.

These pay scales are based on a full-time working week of 37½ hours but individual arrangements are for negotiation between the nurse and her employer.

Other conditions of service to be discussed should include:

1   Hours of duty
2   Provision of uniform
3   Annual leave. In the NHS for the above grades it would be five weeks, exclusive of the statutory and public holidays

4   Sick pay allowance
5   Pension scheme
6   Period of notice
7   Professional fees (e.g. membership of the RCN).

Pension scheme

Any professional person who is in employment which does not automatically guarantee a pension (e.g. full-time in the NHS) should give thought to the provision of a private pension scheme. There are many of these available which give a varying return, depending on the size of the premium and the length of time to retirement. For nurses who intend to stay with a practice for many years and who are working between half- and full-time, it is worth making enquiries about the various schemes available. Many well-known insurance companies arrange these and details can be obtained from the practice accountant or from advertisements in journals and newspapers. The premiums are tax allowable and it would seem reasonable for an employer to provide a private pension scheme for a nurse who had been working with him or her for several years and obviously intended to do so until retirement. This is a matter for individual negotiation but many practices would see this as a reasonable request from the employer's point of view. In those cases where the request is refused the nurse should give thought to taking out her own private pension scheme, as this is worth the cost even over a comparatively short contributing period before retirement, such as ten years.

FURTHER READING

Pyne Reginald H. (1981) *Professional Discipline in Nursing. Theory and Practice.* Blackwell Scientific Publications, Oxford.
The Royal College of Nursing Members Handbook and their publications:
  Guidelines on Confidentiality in Nursing.
  Drug Administration—A Nursing Responsibility.
  The Extended Clinical Role of the Nurse.
Dimond B. (1988) Health and safety issues. *Practice Nurse Journal,* **1**, pp. 108–112, July/Aug.

Chapter 14

Research and Teaching

Any new discipline has to establish itself by identifying and exploring the areas peculiar to it. The rapid expansion of practice nurse numbers over the past ten years has led to many new ideas and role perceptions and these need to be developed. Research explores these boundaries and teaching establishes the body of knowledge required to practise the discipline.

RESEARCH

Until very recently most research into the work of practice nurses had been done by doctors and related to the type of activities undertaken by nurses working in general practice. These basic studies were required to obtain background information and it was the publications of research workers such as Reedy[1] and Bowling[2] which first began to identify the impact that practice nurses would have on the primary health care team. However, more recently nurses themselves have begun to publish research broadening the areas of their discipline. Leading the field has been Stilwell who has widely investigated the potential of the nurse practitioner and related her findings to the present and possible future roles of the practice nurse[3]. Many nurses will not appreciate the importance of research within the field of the practice nurse as they will think it does not apply to them. In fact this attitude arises from not realising the meaning of the work 'research'.

Research may well be a very academic and exhaustive study based on a university department and these studies will always be necessary to establish the credibility of any discipline. However for many it will first be the questioning of routine procedures which 'have always been done like this' or asking the question 'Why?' in relation to their day to day work.

Audit is very topical in general practice at the moment and so is performance review, which is similar. Audit means measuring what you do having made a prediction about how you *think* you do it. For example, a practice may have a policy to immunise all girls of 12 for rubella, i.e. have a 100% immunisation rate. Taking an audit would involve looking at the records of all 12 year old girls in the practice to see how many had their rubella status recorded. If 100% are immunised then this would be cause for congratulation, but the authors' experience is that things are never as good as you hope and, for example, you might find that only 60% of the girls were immunised. Again there is no point in doing this exercise unless the practice is prepared to act on the findings and take steps to see that their immunisation rate is the 100% which they had hoped for. Thus having found that the rate is 60% the areas of deficiency need to be identified, the defaulters chased and the audit exercise repeated in, say, a year to see if the rate has improved.

Many nurses would see the above activity as very appropriate to their working lives and a useful measure of their policy's effectiveness in a particular area.

In the clinical field a simple study of two treatments for leg ulcers would determine which was the more effective and would be an example of trying to answer the question 'Why do I do this and would it be better to do that?'

None of this simple research is beyond the capabilities of any practice nurse provided she thinks about her work and is prepared to question established routines.

On recent courses in Exeter the nurses involved have produced excellent reports from their own working activities on such subjects as:

1 Setting up a diabetic clinic in general practice.
2 Audit of the uptake of tetanus vaccination.
3 The introduction of health education activities in the waiting room.
4 A review of the cervical cytology uptake rate in a practice.
5 The setting up of a practice information card getting the consumer point of view.
6 The prescribing of benzodiazepines in a practice.

It is beyond the scope of this book to give detailed advice on research activities, more to wet the appetite and demonstrate the scope of opportunism.

However there are some cardinal rules to be followed if worthwhile results are to be achieved.

1 Identify the question you wish to answer and write it down. In formal research this is known as *stating your hypothesis*. In the example quoted above the hypothesis would be that all girls in the practice had been vaccinated against rubella.

2   Think through how you would go about answering the question and write it down. This is called the *protocol*.
3   *Share your ideas* with someone else, preferably someone able to give you impartial and constructive advice. The partners in the practice may not be the best people to do this although, of course, you will have to seek their agreement before undertaking the study.
4   If a questionnaire is involved get help in designing it and then try it out on a few people to see if the questions you are asking are unambiguous and provide the answers you are seeking. Most questionnaires need some revision after this *pilot survey*.
5   Don't try and obtain too much information without adequate means of analysing it. The collection and statistical analysis of data is very complex and in a large study would require expert help. In a small study in a practice this might not be so important but it is very tempting to think 'while I'm asking this I'll just ask that' and finish up with so much data that nothing is ever done with it! Keep your data collection *simple* and if in doubt refer back to your original question to see if it is *relevant* to that.
6   Do something with your study after all the effort. This may range from first having a discussion with the other members of the practice team about possible changes in policy, or may be writing a paper to give at a conference. The important principle is not to keep it to yourself and waste the effort which has been made. You will learn many lessons from undertaking simple research activities and hopefully be stimulated to have another 'go'.

TEACHING

As the number of practice nurses has grown their need for training has become clear. All of the early practice nurses will have found themselves in the job, often by accident, and quite unprepared for their role. The background of all nurses is the same, training in a general hospital. As with general practitioners, being trained in a hospital does not prepare them for many of the problems they will have to face in primary care. The training of practice nurses and the problems they face have been exactly parallelled in general medical practice in the past thirty years.

The first reported training courses were organised by general practitioners who recognised the need of nurses to have more formal training for their new role. However most nurses still learnt by being dropped in at the deep end and encouraged to survive!

Fortunately things are changing and English Nursing Board (ENB) approved courses are springing up all over the country to meet the needs of those nurses joining this branch of the profession or expanding the knowledge of those already in it. The involvement of the ENB in approving recognised training courses is to be welcomed as it places the recognition of practice nurses' education on a professional footing. The ENB has been involved in exploring the educational needs of the practice nurse since the report of the joint working party on Training needs of practice nurses[4] (1984) which reported in detail the specific areas to be covered in training practice nurses. The ENB assesses the suitability of courses for recognised training following the guidelines published in that report.

A number of different types of course are now available for practice nurses. These include training courses, study days and specialist courses.

Basic courses

These are usually between one and two weeks in length and can be organised in residential modules, a series of day release or a mixture of both. They usually offer a wide variety of subjects of relevance, particularly to those who have been practice nurses for perhaps a year or two. Certificates of attendance may be offered and will become more common as inevitably some paper qualification will be required as regulations and qualifications become more formalised under the guidance of the ENB.[5] It is likely that training will eventually lead to a postgraduate diploma or equivalent.

Topics covered might include:

1   The role of the primary health care team.
2   Emergencies.
3   Minor ailments.
4   Treatment room organisation.
5   Taking and reading ECGs.
6   Project work.
7   Contraception.
8   Infectious diseases.
9   The use of the laboratory.
10 Chronic conditions e.g. asthma and hypertension.

Hopefully the course would be organised in such a way as to allow active participation from the nurses in group work and discussion, plus the encouragement to do some practical work based within their own setting.

Study days

Many local practice nurse groups have now developed throughout the country and have begun to meet their own educational needs by organising study days, often in conjunction with the local postgraduate centre and the GP course organisers and clinical tutors. The content and format of these will vary according to the local need but they serve a valuable purpose in keeping nurses up-to-date with the topics plus giving them an opportunity to meet and discuss issues with their peers. The latter is a particularly vital part of all continuing education activities as it is very easy for practice nurses to become isolated and not have the opportunity to develop professionally if they do not meet their peers in this way.

Specialist courses

Some enthusiasts have established courses to meet a particular need. A good example of this can be found in the Asthma Training Centre where two or three day courses enable nurses to become expert at the day to day management of asthma and the advice to give to patients concerning the disease and the many different types of inhaler and nebuliser used in treatment. Details of all these types of course can be found via local groups, advertisements in the local postgraduate centres and advertisements in the national press, especially as practice nurses now have their own journal.

The funding of courses

One of the important features which has handicapped the more rapid development of courses has been the confused situation as regards funding. Until fairly recently courses were only organised by enthusiasts giving freely of their time and the course participants paying out of their own pocket for any expenses incurred.

Practice nurses have always been the 'poor relation' within the guidelines of the 'Red Book'. For many years the receptionists had their conditions for attending courses clearly stated but there was always some ambiguity about the position of nurses in regard to claiming expenses for attending approved courses. This reflects the way the regulations have become outdated and it is a great pity that it has taken so long for the medico-political machinery to attend to these discrepancies. The present position is that practice nurses attending Section 63 approved courses should have 70% of their expenses reimbursed by the local Family Practitioner Committee. If there is any doubt, then enquiries should be made before attending the course to confirm that expenses are reimbursible.

This still leaves the question of fees needed to cover the cost of speakers etc. and for some courses this can be a considerable sum of money. Many practices have paid the fees for their nurses and then claimed these as a practice expense so that it is tax deductible. Those nurses attending courses and not supported by their own doctors have had to pay the fees themselves and in this case the cost is not tax deductable. It is quite wrong that this branch of the profession should be discriminated against in this way as no other group has to bear the full cost of their own training.

Progress is being made slowly. In 1988 £150 000 was released by the DHSS to help fund training for practice nurses. About £100 000 of this was used to support existing ENB approved courses and £50 000 has been set aside to develop distance learning methods, for example, the making of a training video tape on cervical smear screening.

It is likely that regulations will change soon enabling practice nurses to have at least the same funding opportunities as other members of the primary health care team. Until this happens general practitioners should do all that they can to support the training needs of their nurses. After all, it will be the practice which benefits from the extra skills obtained and the expense incurred will be relatively small within the overall practice accounts.

National conference

The final acknowledgement that practice nurses have become a force in their own right has been the success of the national conferences which have attracted nurses from all over the country. At the fifth practice nurse conference held at Exeter University in 1988 there were 350 delegates who over three days debated many issues vigorously ranging from AIDS to nursing politics.[6][7] This is a very healthy sign for the future development of the profession and all practice nurses should try and join a local group and perhaps finally get to a national conference so that professional barriers and isolation are irrevocably broken down to the benefit of the profession as a whole.

It has been the intention of the final chapter of this book to widen the horizon of the nurse working in the practice. The intention has not been to give a detailed description of how to do research or run a course but to encourage every practice nurse to do her bit in becoming involved in the development of this exciting branch of the nursing profession.

REFERENCES

1   Reedy B.L.E.C., Phillips P.R. and Newell D.J. (1976) Nurses and nursing in primary medical care in England. *British Medical Journal*. ii, 1304–1306.
   Reedy B. (1977) *Trends in general practice in The Health Team*. J. Fry (Ed).

Published for the Royal College of General Practitioners by the British Medical Association.

Reedy B. (1978) *The New Health Practitioners in America—A Comparative Study.* King Edward's Hospital Fund for London.

Reedy B.L.E.C Metcalfe A.V., de Roumanie M. and Newell D.J. (1980a) The social and occupational characteristics of attached and employed nurses in general practice. *Journal of the Royal College of General Practitioners* **30**, 477–482.

Reedy B.L.E.C., Stewart T.I. and Quick J.B. (1980) Attachment of a physician's assistant to an English general practice. *British Medical Journal,* **281**, 664–666.

2   Bowling A. (1981) *Delegation in General Practice—A Study of Doctors and Nurses.* Tavistock Publications.

3   Stilwell B. (1985) Prevention and health; the concern of nursing. *Journal of the Royal Society of Health,* **105**, 60–62.

Greenfield S., Stilwell B., Drury M. (1987) Practice nurses: social and occupational characteristics. *Journal of the Royal College of General Practitioners,* **37**, 341–345.

Stilwell B. and Drury M. (1988) Description and evaluation of a course for practice nurses. *Journal of the Royal College of General Practitioners,* May 1988, 203–206.

4   RCN publication (1984) *Training Needs of Practice Nurses.* Oct.

5   Robottom B. (1988) The practice nurse course. *Practice Nurse Journal,* **1**, (2) 88–90.

6   Peachey M. (1988) The challenge of change. *Practice Nurse Journal,* **1**, (1).

7   Bolden S. (1988) Countdown to a conference. *Practice Nurse Journal,* **1**, (5).

Appendix I

PRESCRIPTION FOR MALARIA PROPHYLAXIS

```
Patients Name   .............................................
Patients Address  ........................................
                  ........................................

To the Pharmacy:-
Please Supply:-   1) Tabs. Maloprim-No. of Tabs (      ) 1 Dose Weekly
                  2) Tabs. Chloroquine 300mgms-No. of Tabs (      )
                                          base         1 Dose Weekly
                  3) Tabs. Avloclor-No. of Tabs (      ) 1 Dose Weekly
                  4) Tabs. Paludrine-No. of Tabs (      ) 2 Tabs together
                                                            daily

FOR MALARIA PROPHYLAXIS

START 1 WEEK BEFORE ENTERING INFECTED AREA AND CONTINUE 6 WEEKS
AFTER LEAVING INFECTED AREA.

                        Doctors Signature  ....................
```

Appendix II

PATIENT INSTRUCTION LEAFLET FOR TAKING THE PILL

<u>Instructions for taking the Pill - 21 Day Regime</u>

1) The <u>first</u> course of tablets must begin as follows:-

   On the first day of the period take the first tablet.
   Take one tablet daily for 21 days, then stop for 7 days.
   In the 7 days in which no tablets are taken, menstrual bleeding will
   normally occur. The first period will probably occur a few days earlier
   than expected.

2) After 7 days without tablets begin the next course of 21 tablets and
   continue in this way. You will find that each course of tablets begins
   on the same day of the week.

3) If you forget to take the tablet any night, you should take it the next
   morning or as soon as possible the next day. If you vomit within one
   hour of swallowing the tablet, take another.

4) If you follow these instructions you are protected throughout the cycle,
   including the days between one course of tablets and the next.

5) If slight staining or spotting of blood or any bleeding occurs during a
   course of tablets, carry on taking the tablets.

6) If the expected monthly period does not occur after the tablets are
   stopped - do not worry provided you have taken the tablets as directed.
   Allow 7 clear days, then start the next course of tablets.

7) If you miss two consecutive periods, let the Doctor know.

8) Whenever Medical or Surgical treatment is necessary, please inform the
   Doctor concerned that you are taking the pill.

9) <u>SOME</u> antibiotics and other tablets affect the working of the pill. If
   you are given treatment, please inform the Doctor that you are taking the
   pill.

10) In some instances, if you have diarrhoea and vomiting, the pill is not
    absorbed, so it is advisable to use an extra contraceptive method (the
    sheath) for the remainder of the month and until the next packet of pills
    are commenced.

11) If you have any worries, do not hesitate to contact the Health Centre.

Appendix III

EXAMPLE OF A DEVELOPMENTAL ASSESSMENT CHART

DEVELOPMENT CHART (GM = Gross motor: FM = Fine motor: S = Social: L = Language)

1. Mark "X" for items which child could perform.
2. Mark "O" for items which child could not perform.
3. For items which could not be, or were not tested enter "N.T." instead of "X" or "O".
4. The rectangles give the expected abilities at each age. Where an expected function is not achieved, test abilities higher up the same vertical column.
5. Record Mother's observations and results of Physical Examination in right hand column.
6. Summary: "N" = Normal. "O" = Requires Observation. "AB" = Abnormal, requiring investigation.

	TEST	Actual Age	6/52	3/12	6/12	9/12	12/12	18/12	2 yr.	3 yr.	4 yr.	Physical Examination; Mother's Comments	SUMMARY N	O	AB	
6 weeks	GM	Lifted prone, momentarily holds head in line with body.															DOCTOR
		Lies prone with pelvis flat, hips extended.															
		Pull to sit, head lag partly controlled															
	FM	Hands closed															
		Grasp reflex +															
	S	Smiles at mother															
		Follows objects side to middle															
	L	Single vowels, ah, eh, uh.															
3 months	GM	Lifted prone, holds head up											Hips				DR. OR NURSE
		Lying prone, lifts head 45° — 90°															
		Pull to sit — only slight head lag															
	FM	Hands loosely open															
		Holds rattle momentarily															
	S	Supine, watches own hands															
		Follows objects side to side															
	L	Squeals of pleasure											P.K.U. Blood phenylanine				
6 months	GM	Lying prone, back is extended and weight on hands (not arms)															DR. OR NURSE
		Rolls prone to supine															
		Sits up with hands forward for support															
		Weight bearing on legs															
	FM	Cubes grasped against thenar eminence															
		Transfers cubes from one hand to other															
		Reaches out for objects											Hips				
	S	Alert: responds to mother and examiner															
		Smiles and laughs															
	L	Gurgles and coos															

	DOCTOR	DR. OR NURSE	DR. OR NURSE	DOCTOR

9 months

GM — Sits steadily / Stands up, holding on
FM — Creeps on hands and knees / Crude thumb-finger grasp
S — Waves "bye-bye"
L — Knows his own name

Hearing Responses at 18" (Lt. and Rt.)

	Prompt	Delayed	Nil
Cup and Spoon			
Rattle			
"OOO"			
"PSS"			

Visual Acuity (Stycar Balls)
Squint

12 months

GM — Pivots stably while sitting / Walks — one hand held
FM — Fine pincer grasp = finger/thumb / Throws objects down and watches
S — Plays "Peep-bo" / Responds to simple commands
L — Uses 2 - 3 words with meaning

Hips

18 months

GM — Throws ball without falling / Walks upstairs, one hand held
FM — Builds 3 - 4 cubes / Feeds without rotating spoon
S — Dry by day mostly / Understands simple orders
L — Several intelligible words

2 years

GM — Kicks ball without overbalancing / Walks backward in imitation
FM — Unscrews lids, turns door knobs / Builds 6 - 7 cubes
S — Can put on shoes and socks / Watches others play, but does not join in / Asks for drink, food, toilet
L — Joins 2 or 3 words in sentences

Hearing Responses at 4' (Lt. and Rt.)

	Prompt	Delayed	Nil
Simple commands			
Name spoken			
?'s with pictures			

Visual Acuity (Stycar Toys)
Squint

	DR. OR NURSE	DOCTOR	DOCTOR

3 years

- GM: Can stand on one foot
- Jumps off bottom step
- FM: Builds 9 cubes
- Can dress fully except for buttons
- Draws man on request
- S: Joins in play
- L: Constantly asking questions

4 years

- Hops on one foot
- FM: Can button clothes fully
- Attends to own toilet needs
- Imaginative play
- S: Tells stories
- L: Counts up to Ten
- Questioning at its height

Hearing Responses at 4' (Lt. and Rt.)

	Prompt	Delayed	Nil
Simple commands			
Questions with picture book			

Visual Acuity

Lt.   Rt.

Squint

PRESCHOOL ASSESSMENT AND SUMMARY

Appendix IV

EXAMPLE OF A PERCENTILE CHART

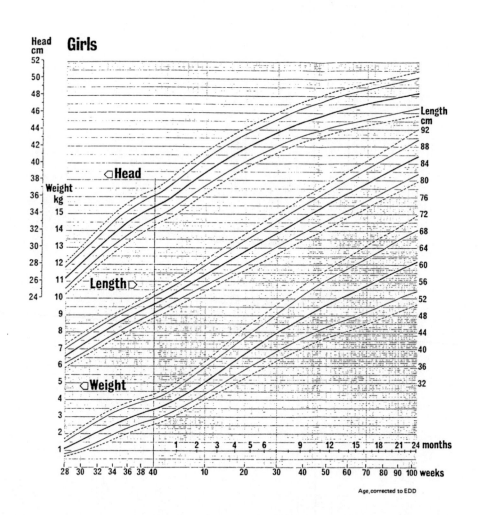

Appendix V

DIABETIC RECORD CARDS

Date																			
Weight																			
Blood Pressure																			
Urine Protein Ketones																			
Blood Sugar																			
Glycosylated HbA1c																			
Creatinine																			
V A (Pinhole) R / L																			
Fundi (dilated) R / L																			
Pulses P. Tib R / L																			
D. Peo R / L																			
Ankle Reflexes R / L																			
Sensation Pin Prick R / L																			
Vibration R / L																			
Treatment																			

REGULAR SCREENING CHART:

HEIGHT: WEIGHT:

TARGET WEIGHT:

Regular screening for complications is essential for most diabetics. Any problems that may arise can then be treated before serious damage occurs.

It would be wise if screening became a yearly habit, in the end only you can take the responsibility for your health.

	YEAR										
1	WEIGHT										
2	ASSESSMENT OF CONTROL e.g. HbA1c										
3	BLOOD PRESSURE										
4	EYES										
	EYE EXAM. with PUPIL DILATED	Rt.									
		Lt.									
	VISION TEST WITH PINHOLE	Rt.									
		Lt.									
5	KIDNEY FUNCTION URINE PROTEIN										
6	SENSATION IN FEET	Rt.									
		Lt.									
7	PULSES IN FEET	Rt.									
		Lt.									
8	INFLUENZA VACCINATION										

YEAR: TARGET WEIGHT: CURRENT DIET/INSULIN/TABLETS

ACTIVE PROBLEMS:

DATE	WEIGHT	Urine glu ket. prot	Bl. glucose Time	PATIENT Urine/ Blood control	TREATMENT	HbA1c	Appt.

ANNUAL REVIEW

EYES: Rt: Lt:

LENS:

VA (Pinhole)

FUNDI (Dilated)

R: L: B.P

PULSES	P.Tib D.Ped		Smokes
REFLEXES	Knee Ankle		Alcohol: units per week
SENS	PP Vibn		Creatinine
			Cholesterol

CONDITION OF FEET:

Appendix VI

DIABETIC DIET INSTRUCTIONS

Guidelines to the new diabetic diet

In all cases diet is a very important part of the treatment for diabetes mellitus. The British Diabetic Association has recently brought out dietary guidelines for diabetics. These guidelines are based on recent research which has been carried out for the treatment of diabetes and suggest the most suitable type of diet for the diabetic patient today.

1) The energy content of the diet should be controlled. It has been found that diabetic control can be affected by varying the calorie content of the diet even when excess calories are not coming from carbohydrate foods. Excess amounts of fatty foods or protein foods can mean poor control for the diabetic patient. The energy content of the diet will vary from patient to patient depending on the individual requirement.

2) For most patients the proportion of fat in the diet should be reduced as excessive amounts of fat have been linked with an increased risk of coronary heart and arterial disease in diabetics. The fat content of the diet can be reduced in a number of ways e.g., using low fat spread instead of butter, using skimmed milk when ever possible, eating cottage cheese instead of hard cheese, eating lean meat instead of fatty meat.

3) Diabetics should include unrefined carbohydrate foods in their diet. This means eating wholemeal bread instead of white, wholemeal biscuits such as bran biscuits instead of the refined biscuits such as Rich Tea biscuits, including wholegrain cereals in the diet e.g., Weetabix, Shredded Wheat, wholemeal pastas and brown rice. Fresh fruit, vegetables especially pulse vegetables should also be included in the diet.

As the diet is calorie controlled and fat has been reduced then the amount of carbohydrate in the diet can usually be increased. This means that the diabetic can eat more of the unrefined carbohydrate foods. It has been found that better diabetic control is achieved by eating unrefined carbohydrate foods as they are absorbed more slowly that the refined sugars and starches and therefore do not cause such a rapid increase in the blood sugar level after a meal.

For the diabetic patient who has to lose weight it is important that carbohydrate foods are permitted. The unrefined carbohydrate foods are filling and help to prevent 'hunger pangs'. It is thought that carbohydrate foods should provide at least half of the daily calorie allowance.

4) The distribution of carbohydrate is important. Meals and snacks should be taken at regular times appropriate to the patient's medication and eating pattern. This helps to prevent high blood sugar levels especially after meals.

5) Dietary Products—These are not essential in the diet. Many contain more calories and/or fat than the equivalent ordinary product. Most do not contain very much roughage and therefore do not encourage the diabetic patient to increase the fibre content of the diet.

The above factors are the main points of the dietary recommendations for the diabetic patient today. As well as improving diabetic control this diet is thought to be a much healthier diet for all members of the family supplying more fibre, vitamins and minerals as well as reducing the fat content of the diet.

Appendix VII

HYPERTENSIVE FLOW CHART

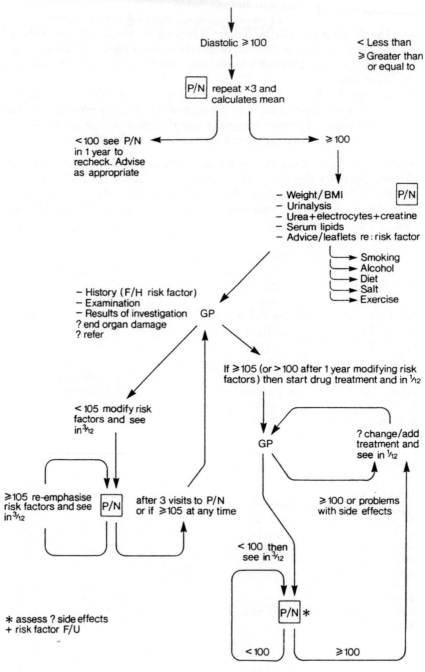

Diastolic ≥ 100

< Less than
≥ Greater than
  or equal to

P/N repeat ×3 and calculates mean

<100 see P/N in 1 year to recheck. Advise as appropriate

≥ 100

P/N
– Weight/BMI
– Urinalysis
– Urea+electrocytes+creatine
– Serum lipids
– Advice/leaflets re : risk factor

→ Smoking
→ Alcohol
→ Diet
→ Salt
→ Exercise

– History (F/H risk factor)
– Examination
– Results of investigation   GP
? end organ damage
? refer

If ≥105 (or >100 after 1 year modifying risk factors) then start drug treatment and in ¹⁄₁₂

< 105 modify risk factors and see in ³⁄₁₂

GP

? change/add treatment and see in ¹⁄₁₂

≥105 re-emphasise risk factors and see in ³⁄₁₂   P/N   after 3 visits to P/N or if ≥105 at any time

≥ 100 or problems with side effects

< 100 then see in ³⁄₁₂

P/N *

* assess ? side effects
+ risk factor F/U

< 100

≥ 100

Appendix VIII

DIET SHEETS

An example diet sheet (reproduced by kind permission of Wander Pharmaceuticals Ltd, 98 The Centre, Feltham, Middlesex).

Each of these menus contains up to 300 calories, so if you take any three menus during each day, that will make a total of 900 calories. Three cups of tea or coffee with a dash of milk will provide a further 100 calories. Vegetables, except for potatoes, peas, rice, broad and baked beans, may be taken as desired. Nothing should be fried. Alcohol should be omitted until weight loss is established; then an occasional glass of dry sherry or wine or spirits may be substituted for the sweet course. Clear soup, grapefruit juice or tomato juice may be taken as a starter before lunch or dinner. If you prefer to devise your own menus, you can use the list of foods overleaf. But remember, unless your doctor advises otherwise, your daily diet should not include more than 1000 calories. But you should eat a similar amount of meat, fish, eggs and cheese as before, and plenty of fresh fruit and greens.

BREAKFAST MENUS

Menu 1
1 glass grapefruit juice (use saccharin for sweetening) 1 rasher grilled bacon (the leaner the better) + 1 egg 'fried' in a non-stick pan + grilled tomatoes 1 crispbread, thinly spread with butter or margarine

Menu 2
2 slices of cold ham + 1 cup milk + saccharin
½ grapefruit

Menu 3
1 cup cereal + 1 cup milk + saccharin
½ grapefruit

Menu 4
2 kipper fillets 1 round dry toast
1 glass grapefruit juice

Menu 5
1 fruit yoghurt 1 small slice rye bread
or
1 crispbread thinly buttered

Menu 6
1 boiled or poached egg
1 round toast, thinly buttered
1 glass orange or grapefruit juice

Menu 7
3 tablespoons porridge (made with water), a little milk + saccharin
4–6 prunes or other stewed fruit sweetened with saccharin

Menu 8
1–2 eggs scrambled with a little
butter or margarine
1 round dry toast

Menu 9
1 cup Swiss muesli + 1 cup milk +
saccharin

Menu 10
Smoked haddock
1 round toast, thinly buttered
½ grapefruit

Menu 11
1 oz Cheddar or similar cheese
1 thinly buttered crispbread
1 apple

Menu 12
1 large grilled sausage + grilled
tomatoes
½ round of toast, thinly buttered

LUNCH MENUS
Menu 1
2 tablespoons cottage pie 1 raw fruit

Menu 2
2 slices any cold meat + salad with oil
and vinegar dressing 1 raw fruit

Menu 3
Filled omlette (cheese, ham,
mushroom, etc.) + green salad

Menu 4
Plain omelette + green salad with oil
and vinegar dressing + 1 raw fruit

Menu 5
Cheese or ham roll, pickled onions
½ pint light ale or lager

Menu 6
½ round ham sandwich 1 glass milk

Menu 7
1 cup (¼ pint) thickened soup
1 roll, thinly buttered

Menu 8
2 plain biscuits 1 pat butter
1 piece of cheese (1 oz) 1 apple

Menu 9
2 Frankfurter or Wiener sausages
sauerkraut or other vegetable
1 raw fruit

Menu 10
1 glass milk shake
2 semi-sweet biscuits (Marie)

Menu 11
Cottage cheese salad (with walnuts,
olives or pineapple if liked)
½ round bread and butter

Menu 12
Crab or lobster or shrimp salad
(up to 1 cup crabmeat) 1 plain wafer
ice

Menu 13
1 hamburger in a roll

DINNER MENUS
Menu 1
1 lamb cutlet + vegetables
1 plain yoghurt

Menu 2
2 slices roast beef + vegetables + 1
boiled or mashed potato Stewed fruit

Menu 3
1 slice of grilled liver + 1 rasher
bacon + vegetables + 1 boiled or
mashed potato 1 tablespoonful
tinned fruit drained of syrup

Menu 4
1 pork chop + apple sauce
2 vegetables 1 raw fruit

Menu 5
Grilled plaice + 2 vegetables
2 plain biscuits + a piece (1 oz)
cheese

Menu 6
Baked cod + 2 vegetables
2 tablespoonfuls jelly

Menu 7
Small grilled chop, small sausage, grilled kidney, tomatoes, mushrooms
No sweet course

Menu 8
2–3 slices chicken or turkey
1 potato + vegetables
1 tablespoonful sorbet ice

Menu 9
2–3 slices duck or goose
small helping of sauce or orange salad
2 vegetables fresh fruit salad

Menu 10
1 cupful stewed meat + vegetables
1 potato Stewed fruit or baked apple

Menu 11
1 cupful curried meat + 1 tablespoon rice
Vegetables Fresh fruit

Menu 12
4 grilled fish fingers 2 vegetables
1 tablespoonful jelly

Menu 13
2 slices boiled ham + small amount parsley sauce 2 vegetables Stewed fruit

Menu 14
2 tablespoonfuls moussaka 2 vegetables No sweet course

Menu 15
1 cupful mince 2 vegetables
Egg custard or junket or plain yoghurt sweetened with saccharine

Menu 16
Steak and kidney pie—about $\frac{2}{3}$ cupful of meat with a small amount of pastry on one side only
2 vegetables 1 raw fruit

Menu 17
Braised or grilled kidneys
1 potato + vegetables
2 plain biscuits + cheese

SNACK MENUS
Menu 1
2 slices smoked salmon + 1 round brown bread and butter

Menu 2
1 slice dry toast + 1 slice grilled cheese

Menu 3
1 slice dry toast + grilled sardines

Menu 4
1 slice dry toast + 2 tablespoonfuls baked beans

Menu 5
1 slice bread with 1 rasher bacon, toasted (toasted bacon sandwich)

Menu 6
1 slice buttered toast + 1 poached egg

Calorific values of common foods

Product	Average portion	Calories per portion	Product	Average portion	Calories per portion
Fruit			Carrots, fresh	3 oz	18
Apples	one	60	canned	3 oz	15
Apricots, fresh	4 oz	32	Cauliflower, fresh,		
stewed without			boiled	4 oz	12
sugar	4 oz	24	Celery, stalk, raw	3 oz	9
canned, sweetened	4 oz	120	Corn, Sweet, fresh,		
dried, raw	2 oz	104	boiled	4 oz	96
cooked without			Cucumbers, fresh	2 oz	6
sugar	4 oz	68	Leeks, leaves	4 oz	28
Bananas	1 (4 oz)	88	Lentils, dried	1½ oz	104
Blackberries, fresh	4 oz	32	Lettuce	¼ oz	1
Cherries, fresh	4 oz	44	Marrow	6 oz	12
Fruit cocktail,			Mushrooms	2 oz	4
canned in syrup	4 oz	108	Onions, fresh,		
Gooseberries,			boiled	4 oz	16
fresh, ripe	4 oz	40	fried	2 oz	202
Grapes, fresh	3 oz	51	Parsnips, fresh	4 oz	64
Grapefruit, fresh			Peas, fresh	4 oz	56
(whole fruit)	½ (4 oz)	12	Peppers, raw	4 oz	30
(juice)	5 oz	55	Potatoes, chips	4 oz	272
Melons	6 oz	24–42	boiled	4 oz	92
Olives, green, in			crisps	1 oz	159
brine	4 (1 oz)	24	roast	4 oz	140
Oranges, fresh	1 (6 oz)	60	Radishes, fresh	2 oz	8
Orange juice	4 oz	44	Spinach, fresh or	4 oz	28
Peaches, fresh	1 (4 oz)	44	canned		
canned, sweetened	4 oz	100	Swedes, boiled	4 oz	20
Pears, fresh	1 (5 oz)	45	Tomatoes, fresh	4 oz	16
canned, sweetened	4 oz	88	Tomato juice	5 oz	25
Pineapple, fresh	4 oz	52	Turnips, fresh and		
canned, sweetened	4 oz	88	greens	3 oz	9
Plums, fresh	2 oz	20			
canned, sweetened	4 oz	88	**Nuts**		
Prunes, stewed			Various, dried	1 oz	156–89
without sugar	4 oz	76	Chestnuts, fresh	2 oz	96
Raisins, dried	1 oz	70			
Raspberries, fresh			**Cereals** and their products		
or stewed without	4 oz	28	Biscuits, plain	2 oz	226
sugar			sweet	2 oz	316
Strawberries, fresh	4 oz	28	Bread (large loaf)	1 slice	65–72
Sultanas	1 oz	71	lightly buttered	1 slice	135
			fried	1 slice	185
Vegetables			Cake, fruit	2 oz	185
Beans, baked	4 oz	104	Cornflakes, Rice		
broad	4 oz	48	Crispies, Shredded		
french or runner	4 oz	8	Wheat,		
haricot, boiled	4 oz	1001	Weetabix	1 oz	100/
Beetroot, boiled	2 oz	26			104
Broccoli, fresh	4 oz	16	Cornflour	1 oz	100
Brussels sprouts	3 oz	15	Custard, made		
Cabbage, fresh,			with milk and	4 oz	128
boiled	4 oz	8	sugar		

Product	Average portion	Calories per portion
Energen rolls, Figgerolls	2	36
Flour, raw	1 oz	100
Macaroni, boiled	1 oz	32
Milk puddings, various	8 oz	320
Oatmeal, raw	1 oz	115
Pastry, shortcrust	2 oz	280
Rice, polished, raw	1 oz	102
Ryvita	2 pieces	68
Spaghetti, canned, with tomato sauce	4 oz	70
Suet pudding	6 oz	630
Trifle	6 oz	258
Yorkshire pudding	4 oz	252

Fats

Product	Average portion	Calories per portion
Lard and suet	$1/4$ oz	65
Mayonnaise	$1/2$ oz	103
Peanut butter	$1/4$ oz	43

Dairy products

Product	Average portion	Calories per portion
Cheese,		
Camembert, Edam	$1\frac{1}{2}$ oz	132
Cheddar	$1\frac{1}{2}$ oz	180
Cottage	$1\frac{1}{2}$ oz	45
Cream	$1\frac{1}{2}$ oz	348
Gorgonzola	$1\frac{1}{2}$ oz	155
Processed	$1\frac{1}{2}$ oz	135
Cream, single	1 oz	62
double	1 oz	131
Eggs, whole	1 (2 oz)	92
fried	1 (2 oz)	136
Milk, pasteurised (1 cup)	6 oz	114
evaporated	1 oz	41
condensed, sweetened	$1/2$ oz	50
dried, skimmed	6 oz	60
Yoghurt (plain), low fat	5 oz	75
(flavoured)	5 oz	120

Meat

Product	Average portion	Calories per portion
Bacon	2 oz	360
gammon	2 oz	252
Beef, sirloin, roast	2 oz	218
(lean only)	2 oz	128
Hamburger, fried	3 oz	312
stewed steak	3 oz	164
corned beef	3 oz	198
Chicken, boiled or roast (joint)	4 oz	216
Duck, roast	4 oz	356
Ham, boiled, lean	2 oz	124
Heart	3 oz	81
Kidneys, stewed	3 oz	135

Product	Average portion	Calories per portion
Lamb or mutton, roast chop, grilled	3 oz	324
roast shoulder	3 oz	300
Liver (ox) fried	4 oz	342
Luncheon meat	4 oz	380
Pork, medium fat leg, roast	3 oz	270
chops, grilled, lean	3 oz	276
Sausages, beef, fried	3 oz	243
black	2 oz	162
breakfast	2 oz	164
pork, fried	4 oz	372
Steak and kidney pie	6 oz	540
Sweetbreads	4 oz	205
Toad-in-the-hole	6 oz	492
Tongue	4 oz	335
Tripe	4 oz	115

Sea Food

Product	Average portion	Calories per portion
Cod, steamed	8 oz	184
fried	8 oz	464
Crab meat	3 oz	108
Eel, stewed	3 oz	318
Fish fingers (three)	3 oz	145
Fish paste	$3/4$ oz	36
Haddock, steamed	6 oz	168
Herring, in vinegar	6 oz	324
Mackerel, boiled	6 oz	234
Pilchards, canned	4 oz	216
Prawns, boiled	4 oz	120
Salmon, steamed	4 oz	216
canned	3 oz	117
Sardines, solids + oils	2 oz	168
solids only	2 oz	120
Shrimps, boiled	4 oz	128
Sole, steamed	4 oz	96
Tuna	3 oz	220

Beverages

Product	Average portion	Calories per portion
Orange, lemon, grapefruit squashes	2 oz	72/78
Bitter lemon, can	$11\frac{1}{2}$ oz	110
Bovril (diluted)	5 oz	5
Chocolate, drinking (made with milk)	5 oz	175
Coffee (half milk, 2 tsp. sugar)	5 oz	115
Coca cola, can	$11\frac{1}{2}$ oz	125
Cocoa powder	$1/2$ oz	64
Coffee	6 oz	6
Horlicks	$1/2$ oz	56
Lucozade	6 oz	114

Product	Average portion	Calories per portion
Ovaltine powder	½ oz	54
Oxo, 1 cube		15
Ribena	2 oz	130
Tea	6 oz	6
Tonic water, can	11½ oz	90
Soups (packet)		
Thick	10 oz	90–200
Clear	10 oz	40–65
Alcohol (1 g = 1.75 g carbohydrate)		
Beer, 1 pint	1 pt	160–220
Cider	10 oz	110
Liqueurs		65–90
Port	2 oz	86
Sherry, dry	2 oz	66
sweet	2 oz	76
Spirits	1 oz	63
Stout	10 oz	100
Wines, white	4 oz	84–102
red	4 oz	72–80

Your weight record

Your weight now is

Your target weight is

Week	date	weight
1		
2		
3		
4		
5		
6		
7		
8		
9		
10		
11		
12		

Appendix IX

CARE OF SCHIZOPHRENIC PATIENTS IN THE COMMUNITY

A written plan of care for practice sisters working in a general-practice treatment-room—three-partner practice in Exeter*

Schizophrenia now occurs in about one in a hundred of the population and is often controllable by chemical drugs of the phenothiazine group particularly fluphenzine (Modecate) or flupenthixol (Depixol) which is a slow-release preparation.

Aim

The aim is to maintain the patient at home and out of hospital.

Doses

If starting fluphenazine (Modecate) for the first time, the test dose of 0.5 ml (25 mg per ml) should be given. The effects normally last between 15 and 40 days. Seeing all patients every three weeks is a reasonably regular routine but the patient's own doctor is responsible for deciding the exact frequency.
    Prescriptions will be written as:

(a)   Inj. fluphenazine (Modecate) 25 mg every three weeks. Mitte 10
(b)   Inj. flupenthixol (Depixol) 20 mg every three weeks. Mitte 10

Precautions

Precautions should be taken about side-effects if key organs like the liver, heart or kidneys are failing. Not to be used in pregnancy.

*Reproduced with permission from Jones R.V.H., Bolden K.J., Gray D.J.P.S., Hali M.S.H. (1982) *Running a Practice*. Croom Helm, London.

Side-effects

Side-effects are the anti-cholinergic group and include drowsiness, lethargy, blurred vision, dry mouth, constipation, mild hypotension and Parkinsonian symptoms such as twitching or stiffness of muscles.

Care in the treatment room

1　Ensure that each patient on fluphenazine has a card which never leaves the sister's box. Schizophrenic relapse occurs quickly once treatment is stopped so failure to attend means a follow-up appointment should be sent immediately and attendance is then checked by the sister.
2　Give patients time in the consultation to talk about themselves and look particularly for the classic features of schizophrenia which are:

    (a)　muddled thinking
    (b)　funny moods, i.e. too happy or too sad in relation to their situation or just not reacting emotionally
    (c)　unreasonable suspiciousness (paranoia)
    (d)　look for side-effects of the drugs especially:
        (i)　Odd movements of the tongue.
        (ii)　Stiffness or twitching muscles especially the face.
        (iii)　Odd movements in general.

3　Ensure patient is seen by his own doctor at least every six months and at the same consultation if any of the above symptoms are present or if the sister just feels something is wrong.
4　Test urine once a year and record.
5　Take blood once a year—usually in the month of the patient's birthday for:

    (a)　liver function
    (b)　blood urea.

Procyclidine 5 mg (Kemadrin)

Procyclidine is used as an anti-Parkinsonian agent and is therefore often used with drugs like fluphenazine (Modecate) to counteract the tendency that these drugs have to produce Parkinsonism.

All doctors in the practice are now trying to reduce the prescriptions for this in order to avoid side-effects from the main drug being masked and will discuss this with any patient who queries the treatment.

Appendix X

CYSTITIS ADVICE TO PATIENTS

WHAT IS CYSTITIS?

Inflammation and infection

Cystitis is inflammation of the urinary bladder—the reservoir in which your body collects the urine made by the kidneys. Often it is accompanied by an acute infection which makes the condition worse. It occurs much more in women than in men.

Symptoms

Inflammation of the bladder causes certain symptoms which are all too familiar. Usually there is a frequent, very urgent desire to pass water—but the amount passed may be very small indeed and does not relieve the discomfort. Very often there is a painful, burning sensation during the passage of water. Or there may be a constant dull ache around the lower abdomen. Sometimes there may be blood in the urine, caused by inflammation of the bladder and its outlet tube (the urethra). Occasionally, there is fever, with general body aches and discomfort.

How does Cystitis happen?

The vulnerable bladder

The female bladder is much more vulnerable to inflammation and infection than the male bladder. In the female, the outlet tube (urethra) is very short, and it ends in the vaginal area, quite close to the opening of the bowel (the anus). It is therefore open to irritation from a number of sources and provides an easy route for infection to pass up the bladder. Exposure to cold and wet, or general debility due to illness can lower resistance and increase vulnerability to attacks of cystitis.

Irritation from the outside

External causes of cystitis include anything which is likely to irritate and inflame the opening of the urethra, paving the way for the bladder to become inflamed and infected. Intimate deoderants, scented sprays, highly perfumed soaps, bath essences and vaginal douches are thought to be capable of causing local chemical irritation. Physical irritation may happen during sexual intercourse—but the risk of this can be greatly reduced by special attention to lubrication and personal hygiene.

Infection

Irritation and inflammation lower resistance to infection by bacteria and other germs. Most commonly, bacteria from the bowel are involved in cystitis. These germs pass out in the stools—and may linger in the anal area, which is very close to the opening of the urethra. Naturally, they thrive in a moist, warm environment—the sort of environment which is encouraged by wearing tights and panty hose. Left alone to multiply, they are ready to pass up the urethra and invade the bladder if given the opportunity. Again, personal hygiene can help reduce the risk.

Irritation from inside

Occasionally, irritation may come from the inside. Constant stressing of the bladder by putting off a visit to the toilet is one form of 'irritation'. In some people the urine is more acid than it should be, and this causes irritation. Excessive amounts of strong tea, coffee, alcohol, concentrated fruit juice, raspberries, strawberries and citrus (acid-tasting) fruits—all tend to increase the acidity of the urine.

Refined sugar and sweet foods, hot curries, chilli and other highly spiced foods may also have an irritant effect. However, such internal irritants are very seldom, if ever, the real cause of inflammation. They simply make it worse if it already exists.

How to relieve Cystitis

Medicines from your doctor

Your doctor may prescribe an antibiotic to clear infection—especially if he has tested your urine and found that bacteria are present. Other medicines are used to relieve symptoms mainly making the urine more alkaline (less acid). Even so, there are a number of ways in which you can help yourself—or help the medicines to help you.

Flushing out the bladder

It is very important to empty your bladder properly. So count up to 20 while passing water and make an effort at the end to get rid of the last few drops. If you have any doubt that your bladder is not completely empty, wait for a minute or so and try again. Drinking plenty of liquid gives the kidneys water with which to dilute the acid urine. Plain tap water will probably have a better and quicker effect than any other liquids. Tea or coffee can be soothing—but they must be made very weak. Strong tea, strong coffee and alcohol may only cause further irritation. So drink plenty of plain tap water or dilute beverages.

How to avoid Cystitis

Hygiene

Cystitis sufferers have to be particularly careful about personal hygiene. Pants should be changed at least once a day. It is important to wash the anal and vaginal area carefully after passing stools. Always wipe gently from front to back—away from the vaginal area. Use only plain, cool water—and certainly no strong scented coloured soaps as these will tend to cause irritation. Cleanliness discourages accumulation of the bacteria which lurk around the urethral opening waiting to invade the bladder. For the same reason, sexually active women are advised to wash both before and after intercourse.

Again, plain cool water is recommended. Apart from hygienic value, this will have a soothing effect on any inflammation which may be present. After intercourse it is also advisable to empty the bladder to wash out any germs which may have entered the urethra.

Avoid irritation

Avoid the obvious irritants mentioned earlier. Be cautious with your use of vaginal sprays and deoderants. Beware of strong tea or coffee, concentrated fruit juices and highly spiced foods. If you must wear tights and panty hose— at least try not to wear them all day, every day. Give yourself a regular 'airing' when time and circumstances permit.

Index